THE NAET GUIDE BOOK

The Companion to
"SAY GOOD-BYE TO ILLNESS"

BY
Dr. Devi S. Nambudripad
D.C., L.Ac., R.N., Ph.D.

Published by

Delta Publishing Company
6714 Beach Blvd.
Buena Park, CA 90621
FAX: (714) 523-3068

DEDICATION

This book is dedicated to all the patients

Who call their doctors day after day

To ask many questions

About the Nambudripad's Allergy Elimination program.

ACKNOWLEDGEMENT

I would like to thank a few people who encouraged me to write this book. First of all, I have to acknowledge my thanks to the confused, scared, frustrated NAET patients who called me many times during my office hours and even at night on the emergency line to get their questions answered. When I received almost the same questions from every one that called, I decided to answer them in this book form. This should be read by patients and doctors. This should save some time for both parties.

My special thanks also go to my son Roy and my husband Kris and those who helped me to put my ideas into book form. I would also like to thank my printers who did a great job on printing this book.

First Edition, January 1994

Second Edition, May 1996

Third Edition, September 1998

Fourth Edition, May 1999

Copyright 1999

by

Devi S. Nambudripad, D.C., L.Ac., R.N., Ph.D.

Library of Congress Catalog Number: 99-63658

ISBN:0-9658242-3-3

Printed in U.S.A.

PREFACE

The purpose of this book is to help practitioners who treat their patients with Nambudripad's Allergy Elimination Techniques (NAET) and the patients who undergo the NAET treatments. When the practitioners take the seminars, they seem to understand everything. But when they begin to work with allergic patients, many questions come up. Then, from their busy schedule they have to make time to contact our office or another practitioner who attended the seminar to get their questions answered. Likewise, when patients go through NAET treatments, they also have many questions. Since this is a new method of treatment, patients get confused without understanding the whole procedure. They also are frustrated when they do not get their hundreds of questions answered by their busy practitioners.

This book hopefully will answer most of your questions and help you to go through the treatments easily and happily. The "You may eat section" will help the patient have a few essential items to eat during the 25-hour period. Readers should understand that this list does not give the complete list of food and food products allowable. It is advisable to consume a minimum number of food items during the 25-hour clearing stage. This will help the body to dispense less energy for food digestion and more energy to help clear the blockages of the energy pathways.

For the best and fastest results, patients are encouraged to get treatments in the order of allergens specified in this book. Before the patients come to the practitioner's office, they can look up the next prospective item for the treatment and plan the life-style for the next 25 hours. This way the patients can help themselves get through the treatments with less stress.

Record-keeping is a problem for everybody. But accuracy of record keeping will help the patient to achieve maximum results in a short period of time. This book is designed to help the patient and the practitioner keep better treatment records with less effort. This book can replace the runner file in the office. Practitioners can keep one book for each patient and mark the treatments and results in the book. The patient can keep another book for himself or herself, and he/she can have a personal journal about his/her treatments.

Patients are encouraged to read "Say good-bye To Illness" prior to starting NAET treatments with their practitioner. This book will give you some understanding about allergies, allergy related diseases, and how a non-invasive, easy to follow, holistic treatment can give you freedom to live again. Many case histories of managing various health problems are given in "Say Good-bye To Illness." Young infants from day five to older patients as old as 94 have been treated with NAET with excellent results. Many so-called incurable problems have been traced to food or environmental allergies and treated with great success.

The current list of the NAET specialists who have completed the NAET Basic and Advanced training and who are qualified to treat with NAET is available from PAIN CLINIC, 6714 BEACH BLVD., BUENA PARK, CA 90621. FAX: (714) 523-3068. Also look up our website: http://www.allergy-naet.com.

If I can somehow lessen the frustration of the patients and the practitioners , and help the patients get well and lead a normal life, my dream is fulfilled.

Devi S. Nambudripad, D.C., L.Ac., R.N., Ph.D.

Buena Park, CA.

May, 1999

THE NAET GUIDE BOOK

COMPANION TO *SAY GOODBYE TO ILLNESS*
BY
DR. DEVI S. NAMBUDRIPAD, D.C., L.Ac., R.N., Ph.D.

This Guide Book has been prepared as a handy practical reference for patients as they go through treatment for various allergies according to Nambudripad's Allergy Elimination Techniques (NAET). We cannot overemphasize the need for complete cooperation between the patient and the doctor in order to achieve the most satisfactory results with the least discomfort, inconvenience or complications.

All patients are expected to read the book "SAY GOOD-BYE TO ILLNESS" before the initial NAET office visit. It is very important for the patient to understand the NAET approach thoroughly before beginning NAET treatments. This book will help you understand all about food and environmental allergies and will answer the most commonly asked questions about allergies.

NAET is not widely known among the medical community or to the public. Because it is a new development in the field of medicine, we do not, as yet, have enough written material on NAET circulating among interested people. As people discover NAET, through friends or books, they may be anxious or fearful due to lack of information, even though it is a non-invasive, gentle allergy elimination technique. My book , "Say Good-bye To Illness," will explain what NAET is all about and what it can do to improve your health. A number of actual case histories, about various allergies and allergy-related illnesses, will give the prospective patient enough confidence and encouragement to try this new technique. Lessening the patient's fear and concern about our allergy elimination treatment will make the patients' and doctors' lives easier while going through the treatment. When you understand the treatment and completely cooperate with the NAET doctor, you can achieve better and faster results.

DOCTOR'S OFFICE

Let's begin our journey with the NAET practitioner's office. The NAET practitioner must take special care to keep his/her office suitable for allergic patients. When the patients find a particular practitioner's office comfortable and safe to be in during the few minutes of treatment, word will spread quickly through the vast allergic community (which is now one of the largest communities, worldwide). Patients will actually begin flying to that office from all over the world. So it is very important for the practitioners to keep their offices as comfortable as possible, if they are seriously going to treat allergic patients with NAET.

The office should be kept clean at all times. The practitioner should try to renovate and refurnish the office with hypoallergenic carpets, paints, chairs, etc. Chemical cleaning agents with strong smells are to be completely avoided. The office should be free from cooking smells, fragrances from flowers, soaps, incense, perspiration and body odors, massage oils, aroma therapy oils (natural, organic or synthetic), herbal extracts and oils, hair sprays, deodorants, etc. Patients with food and environmental allergies are very sensitive to mold, dust, smells from air-conditioning or heating units and vents. Smells from perfume, formaldehyde, newspaper, wall paper, Clorox, bleaches, detergents, fabric softeners, carpet deodorizers, air fresheners, old or fresh paint are devastating for environmentally sick patients. The practitioner must take special care that all of his patients and staff follow the rules carefully. No one should ever wear perfumes or scented hair sprays. Fresh flowers or plants must not be allowed in the office.

The staff and the patients should be instructed not to eat food in the patient waiting areas. Food preparation, brewing coffee, popping popcorn, cooking in the microwave oven, etc. should be prohibited in the office. Air purifier can be used to remove unhealthy smells from the rooms or the whole office. Electric air purifiers can sometimes cause unpleasant reactions in patients with electric or electromagnetic sensitivity. It is not advisable to use such equipment in the presence of sensitive patients. Avoid loud music and loud noises. If there are noisy children among the patients, parents should move them to another room where they can entertain themselves while waiting. Loud noises can irritate environmentally sensitive people. These immune deficient patients can faint or lose control of their equilibrium and muscles in the presence of any smell or loud noise. The receptors for smell and hearing become super sensitive in the environmentally sick person.

BUDDY SYSTEM FOR PRACTITIONERS

Practitioners should be encouraged to form a buddy system with other practitioners in their vicinity. If a practitioner cannot find the cause of a flare up condition in a patient, or if he/she needs help with a new case, the buddy system can help. Sometimes two heads are better than one. Please do not be hesitant to ask for help if you need it. No one is perfect, and we all may need help sometimes. After all, our aim is the patient's welfare. We have more than 2000 well qualified NAET practitioners around the country. It is very easy to form small groups in your area. NAET buddy practitioners should make it a point to meet once a week or once a month, to exchange ideas and suggestions. Whenever anyone comes up with a new useful idea, please share it with Nambudripad's Allergy Elimination Group family, also known as Nambudripad's Allergy Research Foundation or "N.A R F."

CLEARING PRACTITIONER'S ALLERGIES

It is imperative that practitioners know they must clear their own allergies as soon as possible. They may have a parallel weakness to the patients' allergen. When the practitioner is free of his allergies, his energy system is balanced and refined. In that way he is more effective using muscle response testing with allergic patients. The practitioner must be proficient in his/her muscle response testing ability since NAET depends on MRT to determine allergies and plan the appropriate treatments.

NAMBUDRIPAD'S ALLERGY RESEARCH FOUNDATION OR N.A.R.F.

Our nonprofit foundation, N.A.R.F. is dedicated to further investigation and research in NAET. The Foundation sends out a bimonthly newsletter (6 issues/year) to members for a subscription fee of $36.00 per year. We publish all new developments in the field of NAET. The Foundation holds an annual NAET symposium. All trained NAET practitioners are invited to participate at the symposium to learn from one another. NARF has a web-site. NAET practitioners who have completed the advanced NAET training and have satisfied the training requirement of NARF will be listed on the site. If the practitioner would like to advertise through the site, a single page can be purchased through NARF for a nominal fee. To get information about membership to the Foundation, web-site or the newsletter, please write to:

NARF NEWSLETTER

6732 BEACH BLVD.

BUENA PARK, CA 90621

(Phone): (714) 523- 8900 / 523-3500

FAX: (714) 523-3068.

Web-site: naet.com/ email: naet@earthlink.net

SUPPORT GROUP FOR PATIENTS

It is a good idea to form a support group for the allergic patients. Encourage the patients who are beginning to get well, and are on the way to recovery, to form a support group among themselves. With permission their telephone numbers can be made available to the newer patients. If new patients experience any unpleasant allergic reactions during treatments they can talk and give moral support to one another.

Family and friends are encouraged to get involved with the patient's treatment. Most patients suffer from unpleasant reactions while they go through the first few treatments. It is very important to maintain the patient's spirit during this time, any support will help. If someone has no family, they should at least have a friend help him/her to help through the initial days of treatment. Some severely allergic patients can experience unpleasant reaction anywhere from few hours to 25-30 hours after the treatment. It will be comforting for the patient to talk to a supportive person during those hours. A patients' support group can help in these situations.

NORMAL REACTION AFTER TREATMENTS

Is there a "normal" reaction after a successful NAET treatment during the first 25-hour period? Some patients experience no changes with their first NAET treatments. A few patients find the changes to be very subtle. Others may experience one or more symptoms from the list given below. Anything you notice, other than being pain-free, with an overall sense of well being mentally and physically, is a reaction. The intensity of the reactions during the first 25-hour period depends on many factors, such as the duration of the illness, intensity of the illness, and the status of the immune system.

PHYSICAL SYMPTOMS EXPERIENCED BY ALLERGIC PATIENTS

♦ High/low energy, extreme fatigue, sleepiness, insomnia, restlessness, general body ache.

♦ Sensation of: Tingling anywhere in the body, electricity in the body, movement in the body, temperature variation.

♦ Pain: shooting, dull, distended, pin prick sensation, tightness in the chest.

♦ Hyperacidity, abdominal bloating, belching, hiccups.

♦ Sensation of dust-like particles in the lungs, sneezing, coughing, tearing, post nasal drip.

♦ Palpitation, cardiac arrhythmia, increased blood pressure, decreased or increased heart rates, paroxysmal tachycardia, sudden venous congestion or varicose vein.

♦ Excessive or low libido.

EMOTIONAL SYMPTOMS

♦ Anxiety, nervousness, butterfly sensation in the stomach, depression, mood swings, crying spells, obsession, suicidal thoughts, laughing spells.

♦ Blurred vision, choking, throat constriction, headaches, nausea, ringing in the ears, sensations of hairlike particles in the eye and numbness.

♦ Diarrhea, constipation, itching in the private areas of the body in either sex, impotency, low libido.

♦ Craving: salt, sugar, spices, sour things, coffee, popcorn, sweet smells (flowers or perfumes), chemical smells (bleach), smell of sweat, etc.

One patient carried her husband's sweaty shirt during the 25-hour-meridian-time after treatment and smelled it often to keep her from getting depressed.

Most of the time, if you experience one or more symptoms from the list of physical symptoms, NAET treatment at the spinal level is adequate along with acupressure/acupuncture at the gate points. If the patient experiences any symptoms from the list of emotional symptoms, emotional components also should be checked and treated.

Occasionally a patient may experience the symptoms immediately or within the twenty-minute waiting period in the doctor's office. If that happens, the patient is advised to inform the doctor immediately. The doctor can administer further treatments as needed before he/she leaves the office. In some cases, it may take many hours for the patient to experience unpleasant symptoms. Some patients have gone as long as 23 ½ hours before they experienced any unpleasant symptoms. They may have to suffer the symptoms until they return to the office, unless they have been taught to balance their own body, in order to reduce or eliminate unpleasant symptoms. "LIVING PAIN FREE" with acupressure, by this author, may be helpful to learn self balancing techniques. This book is available at many book stores and through Delta publishing Co. Check the resources at the back).

COMMONLY SEEN REACTIONS DURING NAET

While going through NAET, patients can respond in many ways:

Group 1. These are the patients who feel great relief immediately after their first NAET treatment and continue to feel good. They may be presently sick and allergic to many items, but have found a way to maintain a strong immune system. When the body is clean, without many toxins in the system, NAET treatments are easier and faster. It is advisable to go through some cleansing program when you suffer from severe allergic reactions. For example, taking immune system stimulants, going through effective detoxifying program: liver cleansing, colon cleansing with herbal products, homeopathic products; limiting the variety of food intake, juice fast, allergy shots, colonics, and vigorous exercises are things to consider.

Incorporating yoga and meditation practices, regular chiropractic or acupuncture treatments, enzyme therapy, vitamins, mineral or herbal supplements, etc. into one's life-style on a regular basis will have beneficial effects.

The liver - our garbage disposal, gets overloaded with accumulated toxins. Toxins, under pressure, will convert into heat and circulate in the body. The trapped heat will cause blockages in various parts of the energy channels giving rise to various health problems. The symptoms will be directly related to the area that is being blocked. If the lung energy channel is blocked, the patient can suffer from respiratory disorders like bronchitis, asthma, etc. If the colon energy channel is blocked, the patient can suffer from constipation, diarrhea, eczema, skin disorders, etc. The unwanted heat cannot get out of the body without some help. Chiropractic manipulations, acupuncture, a liquid or water fast, exercise, sauna, cleansing programs, detoxifying programs, etc., can create a port for the trapped toxic heat to exit the body. Regularly done, any of the above programs will release the toxic heat as soon as it is produced.

Group 2. These patients may feel good soon after the treatment, however, as the hours go by they may begin to experience tiredness. Some patients can sleep through 25 hours. People in this group can take as long as 35-40 hours to pass a treatment. When they complete the hours, they usually feel better.

Group 3. This group of people may not feel good soon after the treatment, but as the hours go by they get better and towards 25 hours they feel great. 1 capsule of "Vitality formula" following each meal after clearing the allergy will be helpful (available from Lotus Herbs, Inc.).

Group 4. Patients from this group may experience a roller coaster effect. Initially, they may experience very slight or no improvements at all. They may have a few good hours in a day once they have gone through five to ten basic treatments. Gradually, as they receive more treatments they will have more good hours of relief. Eventually the number of good days will outnumber the bad days, until finally, they experience all good hours and days.

These patients fall into the immune deficiency disorder group, suffering from long standing chronic illnesses or a low immune system, and may need to be treated with many combinations.

Group 5. Patients from this group may have suffered from many emotional traumas and various types of abuses since childhood. Continuous emotional traumas may have caused the immune system to weaken. The poor immune system will lead them to physical and chemical reactions as well. As the immune system becomes weak, patients will begin to react to all substances around them. They need to be treated and cleared physically for basic allergens to strengthen their immune system. Along with the basic treatments, they should also receive emotional clearance for their traumas. Some suffer from painful flashbacks, even becoming suicidal at times. Such patients should also receive professional psychological counselling along with NAET regular treatments and NAET emotional treatments. They will need continuous emotional support for a long time even after completion of NAET. NAET specialists are not trained mental health specialists (psychologists or psychiatrists). NAET specialists are trained to unblock the obstructed emotions in connections with food and environmental substances. During the NAET treatments for emotional conditions, the normal flow of energy through the emotional parts of the energy meridians will be reestablished. Because of the normal energy flow patients will feel better. But we should remember that mentally or emotionally sick people have their weaknesses in the emotional parts of the energy meridians. The emotions are also transmitted through certain physical areas of the nerve fibers. If these segments of the nerve fibers are weak, repeated reactions can affect these areas and the emotional reactions can repeatedly take place until the area gets stronger. Emotionally hypersensitive people should take nerve strengthening supplements for a long time along with emotional support (Counselling). This group will also require combination treatments with the allergen and brain tissue or different parts of brain. Please check with your practitioner for more information. These patients will need large amounts of supplements of B Complex, minerals, amino-acid, L-Glutamine, phenylalanine, and tyrosine after clearing the allergy. The herbal preparation "Bupleurum and Dragon Bone Formula" 1 X 3 after meals, is very effective in mild to moderate cases (available from Lotus Herbs, Inc.).

NAET emotional treatments are very effective when the patient shows emotional blockages along with food and other substances. There are other holistic emotional treatments you can get along with NAET. They are "Neuro Emotional Techniques" (NET, check the Resources at the back) and "La Chance Release Techniques." If you suffer from severe emotional blockages, you may consider the care of a psychiatrist during this release method and, if necessary, non-allergic herbal or prescription medication should be used to control depression, severe mood swings, unpleasant or frightening flashbacks. The NAET practitioner can test each supplement or medication for allergy. If necessary, the patient should be treated for the medicine before taking it. You will be able to go through NAET faster and easier by keeping their symptoms under control.

DAILY LOG

Patients are encouraged to maintain a daily log of all the different foods they are eating, any and all symptoms they are experiencing, all the places and people they are visiting. All other activities and events, especially if there is an unusual one, (new visitor to the family, death or accidents in the family, divorce or any unhappy events, any newborn and new additions to the family) are to be noted. After two or three successful NAET treatments, it is suggested that patients eat only foods which they have been treated for and have passed.

WHAT IS A SUCCESSFUL NAET TREATMENT?

The patient is rechecked with MRT, (Muscle Response Testing) for the allergen 25 hours or more after the NAET treatment. The patient's indicator muscle should test very strong in the presence of the treated allergen. This strong response is called a successful treatment. For example, 25 hours after the first treatment of "egg mix," if the indicator muscle tests very strong, we can assume that about 80-90% of the allergy to the egg mix (egg white, egg yolk and chicken) is gone and it is safe to use the product. With the first treatment to a complex food item like "egg mix," one will not get 100% freedom from that allergy. Because egg has many nutrients, it is not easy to clear all the nutrients in one treatment. The rest of the remaining 10-20% of the allergy to the egg will clear up when all the basic treatments are completed. Some severely allergic cases may need a few more combination treatments to be able to eat egg freely.

Egg is a good protein and highly reactive item in many people. Egg contains many vitamins and minerals. NAET basic treatments treat all the essential vitamins and minerals along with the particular basic food groups. When the basic treatments are completed, the vitamin-mineral content of the egg will also clear along with the remaining 10-20% of the egg allergy. If the indicator muscle tests slightly mushy, you will need to treat the egg again until you show a strong MRT since the mushy muscle-test shows that only 50-60% of the allergy is gone. You can have an allergic reaction when you eat or use products with 40-50% allergy still left in your body. After the allergy is cleared using NAET (strong MRT), patients should be encouraged to eat a small portion of the food daily for few days. This way the new imprinted memory will stay strong in the brain's memory bank. After satisfactorily consuming the food a few times, it can be added to their daily list. In order to get relief from their symptoms, patients should be encouraged to eat only food groups they have been cleared for (after clearing about 5 food groups).

When you are highly allergic to all the nutrients in food, it is not advisable to eat 100% organic food soon after the NAET treatments. Organic products are very nutritious and complex. It takes more energy to digest and assimilate nutrients from complex nutritious products. Initially for a few weeks or in some cases even months after the treatment, it is better to eat semi-whole grain products, for example, 50% wheat bread, etc. Fruits and vegetables should be cooked before you consume them to avoid reactions. Fruit juices can be heated first and then cooled before you drink them. Cooking helps digestion of food. Gradually, you can train your body to digest the wholesome foods without any adverse reactions. In some cases like Crohn's disease, irritable bowel syndrome, ulcerative colitis, etc., it may take more than a year before uncooked wholesome products can be eaten without any reaction. To avoid pain and discomfort patients with weak digestive tract should eat small fragment meals of well cooked, non-allergic food. Taking "Agastache formula" (Lotus Herbs, Inc.) 1 capsule 15 minutes before meals and "Multizyme" 1X3 after meals (Available from Standard process of So. Calif.) helps digestion.

SURROGATE TREATMENT

Patient and practitioner should be alone in the room when the patient gets an NAET treatment. If the patient is unable to be tested and treated a surrogate can be used.

A third person or animal in the room can steal the treatment from the patient. In such cases, the third person will get better and the patient will get sicker or show no improvement. Small children should not accompany mothers for NAET treatments. If the patient is getting tested or treated through a surrogate, the patient should maintain a constant skin-to-skin contact with the surrogate during testing and treatment. If the patient loses the contact intermittently, the treatment may not work.

Mary, a 30 year-old mother received treatment for 9 months. She was treated for over 62 items. The patient began getting worse day after day instead of getting better. Finally, the desperate practitioner sent her to the author. Tests found her still allergic to all the items she was previously treated for. She was treated again for the first three basic items and she began feeling better. During the fourth treatment, while the treatment was in process, one of the toddlers from the waiting area wandered into the treatment room. I stopped the treatment until the toddler was removed from the room. The patient inquired the reason for the pause while the child was in the room. When she was told that the presence of the third person could steal her treatment, she knew why she had not passed the previous 62 treatments.

Her two-year-old accompanied her to the practitioner's office and ran around in the room or clung to her feet during her visit. Her daughter was very sick with sinusitis, frequent bronchitis and colds when the mother had begun the treatments. After Mary received just a few NAET treatments, the child regained her health rather quickly. In this case, the daughter was being treated through Mary as a surrogate while Mary received no benefit without the practitioner or patient being aware of it.

Patients should learn MRT so they can test the allergy to the items before they buy at the market. They may have treated for all the Basics, yet all of a sudden, can react to eggs, milk, vegetable, fruits, etc. They may not be reacting to the original item here; it may be the pesticide or other chemicals in it. If patients are able to test themselves, they can live life with confidence. After clearing the Basics, and learning to test everything, the chances of getting sick from the allergens are very limited.

Special care may be needed if a patient has a specific problem, like alcoholism, gluten allergy, diabetes, milk allergy, smoking, drugs (Penicillin, chemotherapy drugs, radiation, etc.). Please check with your practitioner for more information.

ALCOHOLISM

Patients with the history of alcoholism, may need repeated treatments on B complex vitamins, especially B12 and Paba. They will need mega doses of vitamin B complex supplementation. Complete all the ten Basics, and yeast before treating the alcohol. They should be checked and treated for emotional components.

Cigarette smoke, drugs, cosmetics, drug addictions, caffeine addiction, etc. can be treated after the ten Basics.

CIGARETTE SMOKE

When you treat for cigarette smoking, inhalation of cigarette smoke while treating the spinal segment is necessary to get the complete treatment. How can you make the smoke sample? Take a 1/2 liter jar with a lid. Place some wet paper or cotton balls in the jar. Fill up the jar with exhaled cigarette smoke and close the lid tight until you are ready to be treated with NAET. While receiving NAET spinal treatment, the patient needs to inhale the smoke, then smell or smoke of cigarettes will not bother you at a future contact.

PERFUME

If you are allergic to perfumes, spray a few drops of different perfumes into a glass container with cotton balls at the bottom. Then treat the same way as you would treat cigarette smoke. Smell from flowers, new fabrics, chemicals, formaldehyde, building materials, paints, paint thinners, nail polish, molds, popcorn, coffee brewing, cooking smell, smell from deep fried oils, spices, herbs, hair products, newspaper, inks, etc. should be treated this way.

CONCRETE, CERAMICS, WOOD, AND BUILDING MATERIALS.

Many people react violently to ceramic cups, knife, knife-handle, mugs, tiles, marbles, concrete floors, driveways, wood furniture, wood work, paints, building materials, etc. Patients suffer from general body aches, joint pains, restlessness, weakness of the knees, ankles, or the whole limb while walking on concrete or tiled surface and frequent falling down on the floors. Samples of the particular allergen should be collected and treated in such cases.

TREATING FOR ATMOSPHERIC CHANGES
HEAT

You can also test the patient for atmospheric changes. Many people have problems in extreme weather. Some people are very sensitive to heat. Some patients suffer from extreme fatigue and irritability during summer time. When the atmosphere begins to cool they feel better. Holding a couple of ounces of hot water in a glass jar can make the sample of heat. They need to avoid contact with any heat during the 25 hours after the treatment.

COLD

Some other people are very sensitive to cold. Place an ice cube in a glass bottle to make a sample of cold. While the patient is holding the bottle in his/her palm making contact with the fingers, treat the patient with NAET. Avoid contact with cold during the 25 hours after the treatment.

HUMIDITY

Some people get sick in humid weather. They can get shortness of breath, asthma, swelling of the body, skin disorders, mental confusion, etc. To make a sample of humidity: Take a 1/2 - litter jar with a narrow mouth and fill the jar half way with boiling water. Feel the steam at the finger tips while receiving NAET.

HIGH ALTITUDE

Some people get shortness of breath in high altitude because the oxygen content of the air is very low and carbon-dioxide is predominant. How do you treat for this problem? Fill up a paper or plastic bag with exhaled air and ask the patient to feel the air with the fingertips while giving NAET.

TREATING FOR CLOUDS

Many people complain various levels of discomfort (migraines, asthma, shortness of breath, joint pains, depression, etc.), when there are lots of clouds in the sky, or before a heavy wind or a storm. Oxygen content of the air falls very low during these episodes making carbon-dioxide more predominant. How do you treat for this problem? Fill up a paper bag or plastic bag with exhaled air and ask the patient to feel the air with the fingertips while giving NAET.

LOW ALTITUDE

Some people react to low altitude, morning ocean breeze, cold fog, etc. Make a sample of cold mist by filling up a jar halfway with ice cubes and have the patient feel the cold vapor with the fingertips while treating with NAET. You may sprinkle few drops of water on the ice to create more cold vapor.

DAMPNESS

Allergy to dampness is one of the major causes of asthma among asthma sufferers. Some people complain of asthma or sinus blockages in the early morning or after waking up. Usually dampness is the cause. Dampness and cold, dampness and mold, dampness and fungus are some variations of dampness that may need to be checked. Use a paper towel wetted with cold water (ice water) to make the sample for dampness.

DRYNESS/ DRY HEAT

Dryness can cause simple dryness of the nostrils, eyes, and skin. It can cause skin disorders (eczema, psoriasis, acne, and itching of the skin) and also asthma. Heat up a piece of paper towel or cloth towel in a micro-wave oven for few seconds and feel the dry heat from the towel while you receive NAET.

DROUGHT

Walking in a windy area especially after taking a shower or bath, or sleeping under a fan can cause headaches, common cold, runny nose, sinus blockage, sore throat, etc. in some people. They are simply allergic to wind. To create wind: Turn the fan on and make the patient feel the air at the fingertips while receiving NAET.

AIR-CONDITIONING

First treat freon, ice, mold, and moving air (use a table fan). Next combine different samples: freon and ice cubes, ice and fan, mold and fan, etc. Then combine all the above samples and turn on a table fan next to the patient to create an air-conditioned atmosphere: Have them hold ice cubes, and the other samples in one hand feeling the breeze from the fan with the fingertips of the other hand while doing NAET.

You cannot create samples of heat and cold in a vial like other allergens. You have to feel actual heat or cold with the fingertips. So you have to have hot water and ice cubes available in the office to treat these items.

EXERCISE AND BODY MOVEMENTS

People can be allergic to exercise and movements: walking, jogging, running, playing tennis, dancing, sailing, rowing, driving in the car, etc. Different movements make sensitive people very sick. Allergy to these movements can be treated through NAET, you can enjoy all the activities you like without any unpleasant reactions. Please check with your NAET practitioner to test you and treat you for your activities if necessary.

INTESTINAL DISORDERS

In the cases of chronic irritable bowel syndrome, Crohn's disease, ulcerative colitis, gluten allergy, etc., treat with the basic ten first. Then treat with starch, spices, fats, dried beans, alcohol, vitamin E, food colors, food additives, gluten, wheat, and other combinations. Treat only one combination at a time. Do not try to treat too many items in one treatment because the patient's condition could get worse. One cup of rice broth before each meal can help with the intestinal pain and discomfort. Patients should be encouraged to save a sample of all the items ingested in a day. The combined food should be treated at the end of the day or the next day. Repeat the procedure every other day for 20-30 days. Since most people eat different food items on different days, various food groups will be treated and reactions to food combining will be eliminated.

DIABETES

Special care is needed in treating diabetes, First treat the basics, add sugar and/or insulin to the basics as combinations. Then, treat liver, gall bladder, pancreas, parasites, glycogen, glucagon, and combinations with sugar. Frequent gall bladder cleansing once every two-three months is advised to prevent any stone formation. If there are any gall stones, they should be removed by natural means. Check for parasite infestation, and seek appropriate treatment if needed. Gall bladder stones and chronic irritation of liver and gall bladder can lead to diabetes. Persica and Rhubarb formula 1X3 times a day after meals can help prevent gall stone formation.

DEPRESSION

Patients with depression, suffer from allergy or a deficiency in brain nutrients. After completing the basic fifteen treatments, check hormones, serotonin, phenylalanine, tyrosine, and glutamine. Treat them alone, then in combination if necessary. After allergy elimination, these items should be supplemented with mega doses for a few months. Please check with your NAET practitioner for information.

YEAST/ CANDIDA

Many people suffer from yeast/ candida problems. Treat them for the basic ten, yeast mix, alcohol, yeast and common combinations, yeast and heavy metals especially mercury, yeast and sugar, yeast and parasites, yeast and bacteria, yeast and daily nutritional supplements, and yeast and mixture of daily food (to eliminate the food combining reactions). After treating for yeast and candida, patient should be placed on good cleansing program for a few weeks.

VIRUS / BACTERIA

Apart from treating for the specific virus (EBV) and/or bacteria (steptococcus, E.Coli) the patient's saliva, urine, other body secretions, and their own blood should be treated with NAET. In severe cases, it is advisable to get a sample of actual bacteria or the infecting organism for faster results. If you can treat the patient with his/her saliva within a few hours of a virus attack, the after effects will be greatly reduced.

AUTO-IMMUNE DISORDERS, BLOOD DISODERS/ HIGH PLATELETS/ LOW WHITE BLOOD CELLS/ LEUKEMIA/ CANCER/ CHRONIC FATIGUE / FIBROMYALGIA/ PAIN DISORDERS/ ARTHRITIS

Treat the basic 30 items from NAET list first. Next treat the food combinations: (breakfast, lunch and dinner) together a few times. Then treat body secretions and blood. Sometimes, body fluids may have to be treated several times at different intervals, (every week, month or so) to get maximum benefit.

FUNGUS/ PARASITES

People who suffer from fungus and parasite infestations need to be treated separately and then in combination with blood, candida, mold, sugar, mercury, virus, bacteria, etc. Check all possible combinations to isolate the one that is causing the problem.

All new patients should be encouraged to get a copy of the book titled, "Living Pain Free with Acupressure" by Devi S. Nambudripad, available at each of the practitioner's office or at the book store. All NAET patients should learn the simple technique to balance the body that is explained on page 58. If you do not understand the technique just by reading, please ask your practitioner to explain it further. This technique is to be used once or twice a day, by NAET patients, to achieve and maintain balance in the body and reduce unpleasant symptoms following any NAET treatment. This book contains acupressure treatment points for over 280 health problems. Temporary symptom relief can be achieved by using these specially designed acupressure points. The book has 133 illustrations with acupressure points marked in colors for most commonly seen health emergencies. This unique and practical book will assist patients in keeping their unpleasant symptoms under control while going through NAET treatments.

NAET practitioners should hold patient education meetings at least once a month to educate patients about NAET treatment programs. Friends and family should be encouraged to attend the meetings. Patients can have support group meetings every so often. The doctor should also get involved with the group.

PREPARATION FOR TREATMENTS

It is recommended that patients shop in advance for the food and other items used during the 25-hour period after the treatment. Food, gloves, mask, distilled water, fabrics etc., are the items one may need during the 25-hour period. Another reason to shop before the treatments is that many times the stores are filled with odors (including cooking odors) that can cause a reaction in sensitive patients making them lose the treatment.

Patient should be encouraged to prepare the appropriate foods before coming for a treatment. Patient should eat some food within an hour of receiving NAET treatment, because the treatment should not be taken on an empty stomach.

Distilled water should be used with the treatments of salt mix, mineral mix, calcium mix and chemicals. When the patient is not treating for anything, he/she should be encouraged to drink a lot of spring water or purified water. Drinking a lot of water (6-8 glasses of water) helps the energy move freely through the energy meridians. One should not drink distilled water continuously because it can deplete the essential minerals from the body.

BASIC TREATMENTS

"What are the basic treatments, and why should you treat them first?" "Can't I treat for my allergy to the cat first?" " Can't I treat my allergy to dust first?" "I don't react to any food. I only want to treat my allergy to the pesticides. Can't I treat that first?" Almost every one asks these questions.

The basic treatments include treatment for the essential nutrients, vitamins, minerals, and those that are needed for the normal physical, physiological and emotional functions of the human body. These nutrients are necessary to maintain a good immune system. NAET is a non-invasive, gentle, energy manipulation treatment. If the immune system is good, the energy can be manipulated with the least effort on the energy system. When you do not have a good immune system, allergic reactions are intensified. When you try to treat a severe allergy without improving the immune system, reactions can be very unpleasant and severe. Sometimes, a sudden shift of energy can cause light headedness or fainting spells. With poor immune conditions, the energy flow could be slow and it may take a number of treatments to clear one allergy. The basic treatments consist of the essential nutrients that boost up the immune system absorbed from the regular food that is eaten every day. When you are allergic to the food or the nutrients in the food, you cannot absorb or assimilate nutrients from the food. Nutrients are absolutely necessary for: normal body functions, growth and development, to repair wear and tear in the body, fight infections and diseases, prevent invasion of foreign energies or bacteria and for proper maintenance of bodily functions. When you are allergic to eggs, milk, fruits, vegetables, or grains, etc., you are also allergic to the nutrients contained in them like proteins, calcium, vitamin C, sugar, B complex, etc. that are needed for various body and enzymatic functions.

Proteins are the most essential factors in our body. Allergy to proteins (eggs) can make one more susceptible to frequent colds, flu-like symptoms, bronchitis, sinusitis, pneumonia, many other infections, asthma, skin problems, hair problems: (poor growth, falling hair, premature gray), breathing problems, digestive disorders, muscle and joint pains, fatigue and weakness of the muscles, poor blood circulation, high cholesterol, high blood pressure, water retention in the tissues, mental or manic disorders, poor memory, poor concentration, headaches, sleep disorders, irritability, and hyperactivity, etc.

Allergy to each nutrient like calcium (milk), vitamin C, B complex, etc., prevents normal body functions and causes damages to the body tissue (please refer to a vitamin book to understand the functions of vitamins in the human body).

When you are treated for all the 30-40 essential basic groups of foods and environmental items, you will begin to assimilate the essential nutrients from the foods being eaten every day. This will build a strong immune system. Sudden occurrences of colds, flu's, pains, and various other health problems including allergic reactions will easily be prevented.

The basic treatments encompass: proteins, calcium, vitamin C, B-complex, sugars, iron, vitamin A, trace minerals, sodium chloride, corn, grains, artificial sweeteners, caffeine group, nuts, spices, fats, yeast group, vegetable proteins (beans), alcohol, gums, gelatin, starches, food colors, food additives, stomach acids, digestive enzymes, hormones, pesticides, parasites, chemicals, fabrics, and bacteria.

Allergies always affect the weakest tissue of a weak area in the body. If someone has a weak lung, the patients' allergies will affect the lung tissue. The patient will suffer from asthma, bronchitis or other respiratory disorders whenever they come in contact with an allergen. During elimination of most of the allergies, while the immune system improves, the presenting symptoms can change.

While being treated for many allergies, a woman with fibromyalgia noticed her general body ache had diminished. For months, any allergen she contacted caused her to have localized pain in her little finger. Her little finger pain was due to excessive toxins in the small bowel. It would be beneficial at this stage to eliminate the accumulated toxins with a few colonics or colon cleansers.

You do not have to be sick or bedridden to have NAET treatments. NAET can be used as a preventive health measure. Clearing the basic allergies helps to lead a normal life. For example: assume you have a minor sensitive-skin disorder. By clearing all the basic allergies your skin will improve. Then one day, you drink a glass of orange juice, and develop rashes and hives all over your body. Immediately, you would know that some foreign substance in the juice caused the rashes. You can take a few drops of the juice and self-treat with NAET. The rashes will disappear in a few minutes and you won't have to go to an emergency room for treatment of hives. If you have never been treated for the basic allergies and severe skin rashes appeared, you would not know which part of the food caused the rashes. You might have to go to the emergency room to get some relief. When you clear all the basic allergies, life becomes a lot easier. That is why I stress the importance of the basic treatments. If possible, every one (sick or not) should be treated for at least the basic ten. Better health can only be achieved through proper nutrients, and "proper nutrients" mean non-allergic nutrients. Better health through the right nutrients can give you a better quality of life for a longer period of time.

ORDER OF TREATMENTS

It is very important to follow the order of treatments as given in the following pages. The items are listed according to priority of importance to the body.

The First item to treat in the NAET program is the Egg Mix (protein), because the human body depends on protein for its normal every day function. Egg protein is as close to a complete protein that our body will recognize. Even if we do not eat eggs, our body recognizes the egg protein, due to the similarities to the human body proteins.

The Second preferred item is Calcium, the next important item for body function. Calcium is necessary for any movement in the body, walking, running, eating, heart beating etc. These require a certain amount of calcium in the blood. If patients are allergic to calcium, they cannot absorb calcium from their food to run daily normal body functions. The result may be fatigue, body aches, muscle aches, constipation, (the colon is unable to relax), hyperactivity, irritability, high blood pressure, inability to calm down and relax, or insomnia, etc.

The Third important item is vitamin C, needed for the growth, development, repairing wear and tear of the cells and tissues, clearing poisons from the blood etc. Vitamin C is a very good antioxidant. After the vitamin C treatment, most fruits and vegetables eaten will be non-reactive. Patients can begin to add more healthy foods into their diet list after treating for vitamin C. Many environmental substances contain vitamin C: grasses, pollen, soaps and detergents with citric acid (lemon scented), strawberry or mint flavored toothpaste, mouthwash, etc. After the Basic treatments, reactions to the environment will be reduced. Vitamin C allergy causes repeated bladder infections, frequent yeast and other infections, poor circulation, skin conditions and digestion, etc.

The Fourth item is B Complex. These vitamins are necessary for various body functions such as enzymatic and nerve functions. In addition to treating the B complex as a group, it may be necessary to treat the individual B vitamins separately. Check each B to see whether it should be treated individually. B vitamins are the food for the nerves. With a starving nervous system we cannot do any work in the body. Sensitivities can occur when our nervous system does not function normally. A good, efficient nervous system is necessary for clear thinking and other brain functions. Allergy to B complex vitamins and malabsorption cause various brain disorders: hyperactivity, attention deficit disorders, autism, restlessness, sleep disorders, depression, addictions to drugs, alcohol, smoking, overeating, skin disorders, body ache, fatigue, etc.

The Fifth item, sugar is necessary for the normal absorption and assimilation of B complex vitamins. B complex vitamins travel in the body from one place to another with the help of sugar molecules. Sugar works as the seeing-eye-dog for the B complex vitamins. If you are allergic to B complex, you can suffer from a malfunctioning nervous system. If you are allergic to sugar, the same thing can happen, because B complex cannot function without sugar. Various nervous disorders, addictions, overeating, sinusitis, susceptibility to frequent infections, alcoholism, smoking, insomnia, fatigue, allergies, hyperactivity, hypersensitivity etc. could be due to an allergy to B complex, sugar or both. After these five major treatments, patients should be encouraged to eat food from these five groups immediately, so they can begin to feel better. Most people begin to see dramatic health changes when they complete the first five treatments.

Iron, vitamin A, mineral mix, salt mix, corn mix and grain mix are the next five items in the basic-ten series. These ten items are important in building-up and maintaining a good immune system. If the patient has a strong immune system, he/she could get through the NAET treatments easier. When you have a weak immune system, he/she may experience some side effects like light-headedness, nausea, lack of energy, etc., during the 25-hour period after the treatment. Experience has shown us that you may get through NAET, with just one treatment per item, if the exact order of treatment is followed.

On occasion, we have seen, someone hurry into doing Corn Mix, Grain Mix or Formaldehyde without completing the first ten items. This patient may take many treatments (anywhere from two to fifteen) on that item, before they can get through the treatment or feel comfortable. In some cases, someone with a strong immune system may be able to get through the treatment, without side effects to any item, even if treated out of order. The doctor should be able to detect who needs to follow the order strictly, through MRT testing. It is all right to treat out of order once testing detects the patient has a good immune system.

Generally, it is advised to complete ten basic treatments before beginning treatments for hormones, thyroid, medications, radiation, chemotherapy drugs and environmental items such as: chemicals, fabrics, pollens, weeds, grasses, insects, formaldehydes, paints, perfumes, animals, etc.

If you follow the order as given in the list of basic allergens, it is possible that the patient will take less number of treatments, since one overlaps another. For example: when treated for vitamin A, most people do not react to beta-carotene, carrots, fish or shellfish mix. If you decide to treat fish mix as a first item, you will consequently have to treat fish mix, shellfish mix, vitamin A and beta-carotene separately.

TREATING FOOD ALLERGY FIRST

People with environmental allergy will also have food allergy. Most of the environmental allergens contain food elements. Grass, weeds, etc. contain vitamin C, vitamin A, minerals, vitamin B, etc. In most cases, when treated for nutrients, their environmental reactions will reduce greatly. It is easy to stay away from grasses, trees and weeds etc., but it is not easy to stay away from food for too long. When treated for nutrients, you can begin to eat nutritious foods and be able to absorb them which will help strengthen the immune system and make the treatments easier.

FREQUENCY OF THE TREATMENTS

NAET requires the patient to stay completely away from the offending allergen for 25 hours after a treatment. This involves careful restriction of the diet during the treatment period for food allergies and regulation of the environment as well. We recommend that you undergo one treatment per week if you are very sick, or your immune system has been lowered by allergies or long term illnesses. If you are fairly healthy, but have many allergies, you may be able to take two treatments per week. Ask your practitioner if you can speed up your treatment sessions. The allergen being treated must be completely desensitized before going on to a new allergen.

If the allergen is not completely desensitized, the patient can get an exacerbation of existing complaints. For example: treating for sugars, the presenting symptoms are skin irritations, eczema, psoriasis, acne etc. If the treatment for sugar is incomplete, the skin condition can get worse. If, by MRT, the practitioner is unable to detect any weakness on the treating allergen at that time, please do not treat another allergen. Instead, wait two days to a week, then repeat the test for that allergen, and with all combinations. The patient should be feeling better by then if the treatment is completed. If the patient is still reactive to the allergen, the practitioner will be able to find it at this time. After a few days' rest, the body will reveal the weakness towards the allergen.

Let's look at this situation. The practitioner could not find any weakness for the particular allergen after testing the patient 25 hours following the initial treatment; however, the patient was not feeling well, or was feeling worse. The reason could be that:

1. The practitioner could be suffering from an allergic reaction. His/her blockage is not allowing the detection of the patient's allergy.

2. The energy of the practitioner or the patient is reversed or switched.

3. The practitioner or the patient is dehydrated or starving for food.

4. The practitioner is not very skilled at MRT.

5. The patient is overpowering the practitioner.

6. The patient is too weak and the practitioner is overpowering the patient.

7. The patient has passed about 90 % of the treatment, and the last 10% is too difficult to detect immediately after 25 hours.

8. Patient has passed the physical and chemical levels. The emotional level needs to be treated again.

9. If the patient is getting treated for a large group (like vitamin B or C, etc.), one or some of the items are not completed.

10. The patient was not cleared for individual items in the combination treatment before he/she was treated for mixed energies. For example: before clearing the basic ten, the practitioner decided to treat an acute reaction to a chocolate chip cookie, because the patient reacted to the cookie on that day and has no

time to treat for the basic ten. In such a case, the practitioner should check the patient for the allergy to the individual items in the cookie, i.e.: flour, sugar, chocolate chip, salt, egg, fat, additives, colors, water, the baking pan, etc. Then do a temporary clearance on each item before he/she performs NAET for the actual cookie. At a later point, when the patient feels better, treat him/her for all the Basic allergens.

11. Patient did not wait for the specified restricted time (usually 25 hours, or as it is detected by the practitioner) before he/she came in contact with the allergen. If the patient comes in contact with the treated allergen before completing the 25 hours, do not panic. He/she should wash his/her hands immediately or rub the palms together for few seconds and give himself/herself a balancing treatment (Page 58 in "Living Pain-Free" book by this author). The practitioner and patient should work together to solve the problem, if the need arises.

When a patient fails a treatment, and for some reason decides to stop the NAET treatments, he/she should not panic. NAET is not a dangerous technique. It does not cause any severe or permanent damage to anyone or any system. It is a mild, gentle, non-invasive, precise, energy manipulation technique.

If the practitioner is successful in removing the energy blockage and establishing the energy flow in the right direction, the result will be great and the patient will get the expected results. If the energy flow did not get established in the right direction during the treatment, the patient will not be adding more blockages to the existing ones. They will still have their blockages as before. The attempt to remove the blockages will make the patient tired or uncomfortable for a short period. For the first few days he/she may not feel very good. If this happens drink 8-10 glasses of non-allergic water daily. The reaction will wear off gradually. In a week or two, the patient will reach his/her pre-NAET condition.

The body is very good in adapting and adjusting to any environment. The body will adapt to normal self as soon as it has adjusted to all the allergies throughout the patient's life before he/she started NAET. But it is very important to drink lots of water. Water enhances the energy flow through the energy pathways.

Some allergens can be contacted in unlikely places. This guide has been prepared to alert unsuspecting patients to some common hideouts for these offending substances. Some of the restrictions for particular items during the 25-hour period may seem inconvenient. The guidelines outlined in this book are suggested to not only simplify, but also to speed up the process by avoiding unintentional contact with the allergen the patient is being treated for.

25-HOUR-MERIDIAN-TIME RESTRICTION

There are 12 major energy pathways (meridians) in the body. Energy molecules take 2 hours to pass through one meridian when there is normal energy flow. During the NAET treatment, the normal energy flow of the particular molecule of the allergen is established through the energy pathways. If the energy molecule can complete its travel without interruption and return to the original starting point in 24-25 hours, the uninterrupted journey of that particular energy is imprinted in the brain as harmless or beneficial energy. The brain will be friendlier towards that energy or item in any future contact with that substance.

Occasionally, the patient may overcome allergy to the treated item in a few minutes, or in a few hours. In the majority of cases it takes 25 hours to clear. In many instances, the patient may still experience severe symptoms even in the case of a minor blockage, until the blockage is cleared with NAET. The practitioner can also find the approximate time needed for clearance through MRT testing.

Depending on the severity of the allergy, it may take 30-40 hours to clear the allergy. If you fall in this group take extra caution for more than 30 hours each time you are treated. We suggest that you adhere to the 25 hours avoidance period all the time. If you cleared in 2 hours or ten hours and still followed the 25 hours restriction, there would be nothing to lose. If you fail the treatment due to negligence (not avoiding the allergen for a good 25 hours or whatever time is needed), you may have to go through the treatment again. That means, making another trip to the doctor, spending more money and another depressing day of avoiding the allergen!

Less allergic or sensitive patients have been known to clear the allergy sooner than 25 hours following treatment. They may be able to touch the item without losing the treatment. If you are a highly allergic patient you should avoid any contact with the allergen during the required time.

Cleansing and flushing of the allergic foods and nutrients from the system takes place after the treatments. This continues for the next 24 to 25 hours following the NAET treatment. I strongly recommend avoiding the allergic group for at least 25 hours following the treatment to achieve the added benefit of cleansing the years' old poison from one's system. Patients who do not observe 25-hour clearance for an allergen, tend to come up with many combination treatments per item later on. If the patient takes good care for 25 hours, he/she will have fewer combinations on the same allergen and less future treatments on other items.

After the 25 hours, the doctor rechecks the patient's response to the allergen with MRT. If the MRT is strong, the patient should use a small amount of the allergen and test the physical response to the allergen. If there is any further adverse reaction, report to the doctor immediately and if necessary repeated treatments on the substance or in combination with other items, should be given.

ANAPHYLAXIS

If someone is severely allergic to the allergen (with the history of anaphylactic shock, etc.), special care should be taken during the treatment. The patient can be tested and treated through a surrogate for the best results. During the treatment, patient should not hold the sample for the usual 15-20 minutes. After passing the treatment, the patient may still be afraid to eat or use the allergen. Please advise the patient to hold the item in his/her palm for a few minutes to an hour to see if there are any adverse reactions in the body. The patient can continue to hold the allergen every day for a few minutes (three-four days consecutively). At the end of the test period, if the outcome is satisfactory, he/she can try to eat or use it. This method is very useful in testing the effectiveness of NAET in patients with extreme reactions to drugs, penicillin, milk, eggs, shell fish, peanuts, or latex products etc., before reintroducing the substances.

TO EAT OR NOT TO EAT - THAT IS THE QUESTION

One of the frequently asked questions is "Must I eat during the 25 hours or can I fast?" NAET treatment may appear to be an easy treatment. But various energy changes and energy rearrangements along the energy meridians are taking place during and after the treatments. Energy rearrangement takes a lot of energy. One can replenish the needed energy from food intake. So, fasting is not recommended after NAET treatments. Eat the minimum number of foods from the recommended list of items. Please avoid too many variations of foods soon after the treatments. Limit the food intake to this limited variety of items. Eat any amount from one or two categories. Different foods or food groups take different levels of energy for digestion. When one eats too many varieties following the treatments, the brain may need to spend more energy digesting the various items. Eating one or two items helps the cleansing process.

The lists of food that can be eaten safely are given in this book after each allergen (in the next few pages). We have given just a few items after each treatment. You may find more items to eat safely after each category of allergen. But please limit the items for your own benefit.

After completion of Basic ten, the patient is advised to collect his/her breakfast items together, lunch items together and dinner items together, and bring them to the office for treatment. This food combining treatment will continue for a couple of weeks. This will reduce the need for combination treatments.

When treating for the environmental items like grass, dust, trees etc., the patient is instructed to bring samples from his/her neighborhood to the office to collect samples of local pollen or dust: on a windy day, leave a flat dish with water in an open area near your house for a couple of days. After the wind settles down, pour the water into a glass bottle and take it to your doctor to treat. Use the sample in the doctor's treatment kit also. This rule can be applied to vegetable mix, household chemicals, vitamin supplements, etc.

Please do not treat children, extremely weak patients, elderly patients, and debilitated patients with more than one item at a time. Plenty of clean, non-allergic water (6-8 glasses /day) should be taken throughout the day. Herbal teas can be taken with all treatments except with vitamin C, B complex, and spices. Salt can be used with all treatments except for salt treatment.

EATING REFINED FOOD

Refined foods should be avoided as much as possible. Eat more allergy-free complex carbohydrates and fresh fruits and vegetables. In the initial stage, cook food well if it is hard to digest. If you are not a vegetarian, eat non-allergic lean meats. Avoid excess fat consumption. Excess fat in the food will slow down the energy circulation through the energy meridians. White rice should be used with B complex, iron, sugar and vitamin E treatments. Brown rice can be used with all other treatments.

HOW ABOUT A JUICE FAST?

Fasting with juices is highly recommended after clearing the Vitamin C group. Extremely weak, tired, chronically sick patients, persons with malabsorption problems, immune deficient patients, patients with cancer, Aids, Chronic Fatigue Syndromes, gastric ulcers, fever, etc. should be drinking lots of juices initially. Juices do not require much energy for digestion. Nutrients from the juices can be assimilated easily. After the patients gain enough strength, they can begin to eat nutritious solid foods and increase roughage. Drink more vegetable juices than fruit juices, which should be limited to one or two glasses daily. When on a juice diet, drink 6-8 glasses of non-allergic clean water also. Water will help the assimilation of nutrients.

FOOD CRAVING DURING TREATMENT

Most of the time, when you are treated for an allergen with NAET, you may experience an unusual craving for that particular item. For example, if you are treated for salt, sugar, or spices, you may crave salt, sugar (ice cream), or spicy food respectively during the 25-hour period. Some people may experience withdrawal symptoms. If they resist the temptation and follow the restriction for the 25-hour period, the craving will subside the next day. That allergen will probably never bother them again for the rest of their lives, unless the items are chemically contaminated.

Soon after a successful completion of treatment, you may crave the particular food for a few days. For example, after finishing treatment for B complex vitamins, you may crave bread and grain products. This is because the long-term allergy has created a huge deficiency of the essential nutrients in your body. The brain simply demands to bring more of the essential nutrients into the body. In such cases the patient may need to take large doses of vitamin or mineral supplements for a certain period. In cases of pain disorders, one may need to take large amount of calcium, magnesium, zinc, phosphorus, etc., for few weeks. The doctor will help to decide the duration and amount of large doses of vitamin/mineral supplementation.

NEED FOR SUPPLEMENTS

After completing the treatment for the essential nutrients (like Calcium, B Complex, Vitamin A, Iron, Vitamin E, trace minerals, mineral supplements and Amino Acids) it may be advisable to take supplements for a few months to reduce the deficiency by assisting the body to recover faster.

People who take appropriate supplements after treatments usually get better faster than people who depend on only food to supplement their needs. You should be careful to check the allergy to the particular vitamin/supplements before taking them. Even though, the patient was treated for vitamins like B Vitamins, C Vitamins, Minerals, Enzymes, etc. he/she can react with various, unusual health problems just by taking allergic products. So each container should be checked for allergy before taking it. Another concern about supplements is the possibility of overdose. After NAET treatments, the body is able to assimilate 80-100% of the nutrients from the products consumed. Check the daily need frequently and adjust the dosage accordingly. An overdose can produce allergy-like symptoms which can be treated with NAET (as an allergy). In case of an overdose, hold the item that is overdosed and repeat the NAET every 10 minutes until the patient feels better.

NAET METHOD TO EVALUATE THE NEED FOR SUPPLEMENTS

This method can be used to determine the adequate dosage of prescription medication, vitamin-mineral supplements, herbal supplements, laxatives, amount of caloric intake, etc.

Find an indicator muscle (Find any strong muscle. Please read "Say Good-bye to Illness," chapter 6 for more information on muscle response testing.)

Have the patient hold one vitamin pill (e.g. B Complex, calcium) in his free hand. Test the indicator muscle.

If weak, then the patient is allergic to the pill. Treat the patient for that pill using NAET, or the patient can go to any NAET practitioner who can eliminate his/her allergies by using NAET.

If his /her indicator muscle is strong in the presence of one pill, add more pills one by one into the patient's hand, until the indicator muscle goes weak. When the arm muscle goes weak, stop adding pills to the hand.

Now count the pills in the hand. The total number in the hand is the total deficiency on that day in the present condition.

This number can be anywhere from 1-2 pills to many thousands depending on the deficiency. For example, in certain nerve disorders, the total amount of Vitamin B complex deficiency can be as high as 20-30 thousand grams.

If the deficiency is 1-6 pills, one may not need to take supplements. Regular balanced meals will provide the requirements.

If the deficiency is more than 6-10 pills (or the amount equals 6-10 times recommended daily dosage (RDA), then one should supplement one pill daily. If the deficiency is calculated in many tens, hundreds, or thousands, supplement the person with 4-6 times the recommended daily dosage of that particular supplement, until the deficiency is taken care of. Never supplement more than 4-6 times the RDA amount on any given day. In case of a huge deficiency, when patient is taking mega-doses of supplements (4-6 times the RDA amount), the supplements should be checked every three days. If you continue to take the supplements in mega-doses after displacing the deficiency, you can easily overdose on the supplements and may experience allergy-like or other unusual symptoms.

When that patient is no longer deficient, he/she can eat a balanced meal or take a multivitamin-mineral supplement. When a patient is no longer allergic to a substance, the body will naturally demonstrate a need for that item. This helps to bring the body to a balance by supplementing the long-term deficiency caused by the allergy. It is essential to supplement appropriately to achieve better and faster results when the allergy is successfully treated. But you must be careful not to overdose with vitamins or drugs. After the NAET treatments, the body will absorb vitamins easily. So daily requirements can decrease even with taking a small dosage of vitamins. If you take too much it can become toxic. Use the same technique to measure the toxicity.

Supplements in mega doses are often needed for a number of months in the following cases: arthritis, fibromyalgia, chronic fatigue, any chronic problems related to allergy, hair loss, constipation, degenerative diseases, cancer, etc.

COMBINATION TREATMENTS

The stomach has strong acids to help break down the food we eat. The intestinal tract produces strong alkaline juices. When the food mixes with the acid, a chemical reaction occurs. The end result of any chemical reaction is a new product and heat. The new product produces new characteristics and thus new energy. One may be allergic to this new product's energy. This reaction can be reproduced by combining the energy of the food and acid. If there is an incompatibility between this new energy and the patients,' it can be demonstrated by muscle testing. If there is a reaction, it can be eliminated the same way as the individual allergen.

Likewise, in advance, we can find the reaction between an allergen and alkalinity and RNA/DNA. Heat is being produced in the body during any chemical process. Sometimes, proper digestive steps do not take place when ice (cold) is consumed. It is necessary to clear the reaction between heat and the food, or cold and the food. In the same way an allergen can react with the organs (allergen and lung, allergen and heart, allergen and brain etc.). Sometimes an allergen can react with female hormones, male hormones, pituitary gland secretion, adrenaline, serotonin, pineal gland, one's blood, sweat, etc.

In cases where an allergy is inherited, you may need many combination treatments to overcome the allergic reactions completely. The possible combinations are allergen and:

• stomach acids, alkalinity of the intestinal juices (Base), RNA, DNA

• heat (salt and heat), cold (freon and cold in case of an allergy to air-conditioning)

• Individual vital organs (stomach, heart, lung, liver, gall bladder, pancreas, small intestine, etc.)

• liver (pesticides and liver)

• pancreas (sugar and pancreas in cases of diabetes)

• kidney (salted nuts and kidney)

• lungs (bacteria and lung in case of lung infection, bronchitis, etc.)

• stomach (garlic bread and stomach tissue in a case with acidity of the stomach after eating garlic bread)

• cotton and urinary bladder (cotton underpants with urinary bladder tissue in a patient with frequent bladder infection, interstitial cystitis, where one is allergic to cotton underpants).

• colon (gluten and colon)

• gall bladder(gall bladder and oils)

• heart (sulfites and heart)

• brain enzymes (serotonin and brain tissue)

• hormones

• emotion

• sugar

• eczema

• hormones and calcium - (in case of osteoporosis)

• hormones and sugar - (in hot flashes)

• hormones and salt - (in P.M.S).

• hormones, sugar and heat - (in hot flashes)

• sugar and spleen - (in sugar craving, fatigue)

• sugar and liver - (in liver headaches)

• sugar and brain tissue - (in brain fog, brain fatigue)

• fats and brain tissue - (in sensation of heaviness in the brain)

• fats, sugar and blood vessels (in high serum triglycerides)

• calcium, fats and blood vessels (in arteriosclerosis)

• bacteria and lung tissue - (in pneumonia)

• proteins and lymph (in edema or water retention in the tissues)

- amino acid and stomach acids - (in hyperactivity, autism)

- amino acid, and digestive enzymes - (in abdominal bloating)

- fats, cold and hormones (in obesity)

- fats and vitamin C - (in obesity)

- vitamin C and blood vessels - (bruising easily, Raynaud's disease)

- cholesterol and blood - (in high serum cholesterol)

- calcium and sugar and proteins - (in scleroderma), etc.

After completing the first 30 groups, it is advisable to collect all the breakfast items together, lunch items together, dinner items together and treat each group separately first, then combine breakfast, lunch and dinner together to remove the reaction seen due to food combining. Many people react by abdominal bloating, poor absorption, etc., when they eat carbohydrate and protein together; yogurt and meat, proteins and fats, etc. NAET treatments on combined multiple foods can easily remove that problem. The patient will be able to eat carbohydrate, proteins, fats and spices all at once and absorb the nutrients from the group without any unpleasant reaction.

EMOTIONAL ALLERGY

Many times, origin of the physical symptoms could be traced back to some unresolved emotional trauma. A woman in her fifties complained of hypoglycemia since childhood. She was found to be very allergic to sugar. When she was treated for sugar with NAET, she cleared her physical and chemical allergy. But her emotional allergy remained the same and her hypoglycemic reaction was exaggerated. She recalled that she was restricted from eating sugar. When she was five years old. Her parents told her sugar was bad for her health. One day, as a gesture of love, a family friend gave her a box full of chocolate bars. As soon as the friend left the house, her mother snatched the box from her and flushed the chocolates down the toilet before she had a chance to eat one. The child felt very bad and cried for a long time. Her mother did not take time to explain the reason for her insensitive behavior. This puzzled the child and left an unhealed wound in her heart and brain. Ever since that event, for 48 years, with each contact of sugar or sugar products, she experienced unpleasant reactions, misdiagnosed as hypoglycemia. When she was treated for this emotional blockage with NAET, she no longer suffered from hypoglycemia.

A young man of 32, tested allergic to almost all food items. After treating for the Basics, he still got sick and complained of nausea after each meal. He tried to eat just a few items which had been absolutely cleared for allergies by NAET and confirmed by MRT. He was tested for emotional blockage by MRT and found he was afraid to eat any food that was tied to his childhood. As he was growing up, his abusive, maniac father abused his mother verbally and physically and often beat her or threw the dishes at her while eating. Watching all these horrible incidents frightened young Jim, who often lost his appetite and went without eating. These unfortunate incidents left deep wounds in his mind in association with foods. When he was treated for his childhood fears, he was able to eat food without getting sick.

Suppose two people were fighting while eating popcorn. One got upset and walked out of the room. The second person was very angry. Without paying attention he kept eating popcorn while thinking of a way to solve his problem or to get back at the other person. In fact, at a later time he may not even remember that he ate popcorn at all. While he was eating popcorn, his brain was stimulated with anger and resentment. That was forgotten; however, the brain was aware of eating popcorn, and it was forced to associate this with anger and resentment. The brain, always watching over our welfare, makes a note of this association. In a future contact with popcorn, the brain will caution him about the previous episode of anger and resentment while he eats popcorn, which can mimic an allergic reaction.

After the successful completion of treatment for an allergen, the physical and nutritional allergy may never return. But the emotional allergy can return any number of times if one is not careful to avoid unpleasant things while eating or cooking.

It is very important to respect food preparation and consumption for better assimilation of the nutrients and to avoid the recurrence of emotional allergies.

DEVELOP GOOD EATING HABITS AND PREVENT EMOTIONAL BLOCKAGES

Avoid eating when under stress. Always have pleasant thoughts while eating and enjoy your food. You can play your favorite music while you eat whether you are eating alone or with your eating partner. When you send the food into your stomach accompanied with feelings of love and happiness, your body and mind will cherish the nutrients with love and happiness which will help the body and mind to grow healthy.

Many people bless the food before they eat. This ritual gives you a chance to clear the mind of all troubled emotions. Fill the mind with a sense of spirituality before eating, avoiding troubled emotions and food associations. Try to eat with people who share pleasant thoughts and make eating a pleasing event. Avoid fights, exchanging unpleasant words, bad news, etc., while eating in order to prevent repeated emotional blockages associated with food.

DIET: NAET patients are encouraged to eat non-allergic food whenever possible. After three or four treatments, you are encouraged to eat strictly non-allergic foods from the groups that have already been treated. After completion of each treatment, add that group or item into your diet. This will help you to get through the rest of the treatments faster with limited unexpected reactions. NAET patients should drink 5-8 glasses a day of clear, non-allergic water.

EXERCISE: Regular exercise is very important to distribute the nutrients evenly in the body. Begin very slowly if you are very sick or haven't exercised recently. Ten minutes of any kind of exercise, twice a day is advisable. If someone feels joint pains or excessively tired after exercising, it is advisable to take 500 milligrams of calcium before you exercise. Drink a large glass of water after exercising to help eliminate the toxins produced from the workout.

MASSAGE: Massages should be taken before the NAET treatment. Therapeutic massages improve circulation and thus help distribute nutrients. Massages help to rid the toxins produced during the treatments. The patient should drink a full glass of water after the massage to help eliminate the impurities produced. Vigorous exercise, massage, swimming, Jacuzzi, extreme hot baths etc., are not advisable after the NAET treatment. Wait at least 6 hours before engaging in any of these activities.

ACUPUNCTURE: Acupuncture is used to balance the body. Traditional acupuncture with many needles, etc., should be given to the patient before NAET. Other kinds of acupuncture treatments are not advisable during the 25 hours after the treatment. Just four, six or eight needles should be used on the balancing points to maintain homeostasis of the body after NAET. Balancing points always remain the same for most people. During the NAET treatment, patients react differently to the needles. Depending on the severity of the ailergens some people feel varying degrees of pain and discomfort at the needle site. Severe reactions can be expected for severe allergens: shooting pain, shock like pain, cramps, pulling like pain, dull and distended pain, red welts, etc., can be found around the needles. Most often the reactions will disappear a few minutes after the needle insertion. If the redness continues beyond 15 minutes, it is advisable to retain the needle for a longer period of time. If the patient feels light headed, or experiences extreme emotional variations like agitation, anger, crying spells, etc., shortly after the stage-1 treatment (spinal treatment) or during the 20 minutes waiting period, the needles should be removed immediately (if they are on needles). Emotional blockages should be checked and treated right away. If the patient is alone or with others in the waiting area and experiences such unusual symptoms, the practitioner should be notified immediately.

After 20 minutes of treatment, if a drop of blood appears when the needle is removed, it is a good response to the treatment. Toxic energy will have a chance to come out of the body through the blood-let area. If there is a red streak, welt or redness around the needle, the needle should be left in for a few more minutes until the reaction diminishes. If there is edema, a black and blue mark, etc., present at the needle site after removing the needle, it denotes that the allergen being treated is a strong one.

Sometimes, the patient can experience various types of energy movements, in different parts of the body, while holding the allergen during the 20 minutes after the stage-1 treatment. If the sensation is too uncomfortable, the patient should not hold the allergen. The allergen can be removed from the palm and placed next to the body.

If the patient reports that he/she tends to get severe allergic reactions to an allergen (history of anaphylaxis) please treat her/him through a surrogate. If someone reacts violently to the allergen, it is not necessary to hold the item in the hand during the stage-2 treatment (needle, acupoint massage, 20 minutes waiting period, etc.). If the patient had a huge bruise, swelling etc. at the site of the needle, if it caused tissue damage in the surrounding area, the doctor should avoid inserting needles at that particular acupuncture point for approximately a week. If there is a hematoma, pain in the needle area, please apply hot moist compresses for a few minutes, it will be resolved shortly. In a day or so the tissue will go back to normal.

CONSIDERATIONS FOR UNUSUAL CONDITIONS

NAET treatment should be avoided in the first three days of menstrual cycle. Acupuncture is not advised during the first three days of menstruation and in pregnant women.

Young children under 15, extremely weak patients, pregnant women, women who are in their first three days of menstrual cycle, patients who are afraid of acupuncture needles, patients with history of acupuncture needle shocks, patient with skin infections, swelling of the limbs, etc., should not be needled. Massages on the acupoints will be sufficient to complete the treatment.

Patients with spinal deformity, severe case of spinal segmental degeneration, moderate to severe scoliosis, severe arthritis, patients with highly sensitive back, recent back surgery, abnormal growths on the spine or on the back, young children under two, etc., should not be treated directly on the back. Use a surrogate in such cases.

RECORD KEEPING

Space is provided in this guidebook for the patient to keep a record of individual treatments and notes of progress.

In addition, pages are provided to help the patient start a food diary and chart exposure to other potential allergens and the appearance of any symptoms. After clearing for the major allergens, you might notice numerous reactions to various simple items. When your body gets rid of severe allergies, other allergies could easily be noticed. By maintaining a diary, the patient is able to help the doctor pick up the next most important item to be treated. These records of the frequency of reaction to certain products along with dates, may prove helpful in uncovering unrecognized allergens.

One patient reacted to anything she ate from her freezer. More investigation proved that she was allergic to the fungus and molds found in the freezer. Another patient's complaints of frequent angina pain, sinus problems, arrhythmia, frequent eye inflammation etc. were completely relieved after treating for fungus. Even though she was not eating frozen foods, every day she would pet her dog who was suffering from some unknown skin problem related to fungus. In this case, the dog was also treated for fungus, and the dog's skin problem improved.

Another patient had a reaction to elm trees since childhood. Since she was not getting better with food treatment, she was treated for elm trees. Her condition worsened with the initial treatment, breaking out in huge hives all over her body. She needed repeated treatments for elm tree for one week. At the end of the week, not only did her skin clear up, most of her other allergies improved.

This guidebook is intended to help patients understand the importance of avoiding contact with the allergen for which they are being treated during the 25 hour period, and to make that process easier for them. In no way do these guidelines replace the advice of the professional carrying out the treatments, and all patients are encouraged to discuss any individual problems thoroughly with their doctor.

CLINIC RULES

Rules may vary from one NAET office to another: however, the following are typical of what you should expect in any office or clinic using these treatments:

1. Please do not wear any perfume, perfumed powder, strong smelling deodorant, hair spray, or after shave when you come to the clinic for treatments.

2. There is no smoking allowed in (or around) the office. Please do not wear clothes that smell like smoke or paint. Other patients could react to these smells.

3. Please wash your hands before and after the treatment. After the treatment, if the patient cannot wash his/her hands, vigorous rubbing of the hands for 30 seconds will be sufficient.

4. Do not exercise for 6 hours after the treatment.

5. Avoid exposure to extreme hot or cold temperature after the treatment.

6. Please take a shower before you come for a treatment.

7. Do not bathe or shower until 6 hours after the treatment.

8. Do not eat or chew gum or candy during treatment.

9. Do not cross your hands or feet during the first 20 minutes after the treatment.

10. Do not read or touch other objects during the 20 minutes following the stage-1 treatment because contact with other substances during this period could cause your treatment to fail.

11. Wear no or minimal jewelry when you come for a treatment.

12. Remember to check with your doctor for the item you treated , after 25 hours, and at least within one week (to make sure you have completed the treatment. If you did not complete the treatment, your existing symptoms may continue for a long time).

13. To insure maximum progress with your treatments maintain your own treatment and food diary.

14. You may need to wear gloves while you get treated for environmental substances: (mineral mix, metals, water, leather, formaldehyde, fabric, wood, mold, etc.). You may need to wear a mask while you get treated for chemical smells, pollens, dust and dust mites, perfumes, etc.

15. Always eat before you come for the treatment. You should not take NAET treatments and acupuncture when you are hungry.

16. Do not eat heavy meals after acupuncture.

17. Drink lots of water after NAET and acupuncture treatments to help cleanse the toxins produced during the treatment.

18. Please do not stop any other treatment you are on: medication, therapy, chiropractic treatments, massages etc. It is good for your body to have a general body massage immediately before the NAET or 6 hours after the NAET treatments. Massages can help to improve the energy flow through the energy pathways. If you are taking lots of vitamins and herbs, or any particular drug, you may continue them as before if you think that they are helping you. But when you get treated for the food containing a particular vitamin, herb, or substance, you may be asked to stop using it for 25 hours following that particular treatment.

19. NAET treatment will not interfere with any other treatment. In fact, if you can keep your presenting symptoms under control with whatever method you are using, NAET treatment will be a lot easier.

PATIENT'S CHART OF MAJOR SYMPTOMS

Before Treatment: Date: Improvements Noticed:

PATIENT'S RECORD OF TREATMENTS

FOOD ITEMS:	Date Treated:	Cleared:
1. Chicken, Egg		
2. Milk /Calcium mix		
3. Vitamin C mix		
4. B Complex Mix		
5. Sugar Mix		
6. Iron mix		
7. Vitamin A		
8. Mineral mix		
9. Salt mix/Chlorides		
10. Corn mix		
11. Grain mix		
12. Yeast Mix/Candida		
13. Art. Sweeteners		
14. Coffee mix		
15. Chocolate		
16. Caffeine		
17. Nut mix 1		
18. Nut mix 2		
19. Spice mix 1		
20. Spice mix 2		
21. Animal fat		
22. Vegetable fats		
23. Amino acid 1		
24. Amino acid 2		
25. Fish mix		
26. Shellfish mix		
27. Whey		
28. Yogurt		
29. Dried Bean mix		
30. Turkey		
31. Whiten-all		

32. Fluoride _____

33. Gelatin _____

34. Alcohol _____

35. Baking powder/Baking Soda _____

36. Gum mix _____

37. Vegetable mix _____

38. Vitamin D _____

39. Vitamin E _____

40. Vitamin K _____

41. Vitamin F _____

42. Vitamin P _____

43. Vitamin T _____

44. RNA/DNA _____

45. Acid _____

46. Base _____

47. PT. _____

48. Serotonin _____

49. Food colorings _____

50. Food additives _____

51. Chromium _____

52. Cobalt _____

53. Copper _____

54. Germanium _____

55. Gold _____

56. Iodine _____

57. Lead _____

58. Magnesium _____

59. Manganese _____

60. Molybdenum _____

61. Phosphorus _____

62. Potassium _____

63. Selenium _____

64. Silver _____

65. Sulfur _____

66. Vanadium _____

67. Zinc _____

68. Soybean Mix _____

69. Lecithin _____

70. Milk Mix _____

71. Cheese Mix _____

72. Tomato Mix _____

73. Onion Mix _____

74. Pepper Mix _____

75. Potato Mix _____

76. Wheat Mix _____

77. Cucumber Mix _____

78. Melon mix _____

79. Modified Starch _____

OTHER ALLERGENS

Egg white _____

Egg yolk _____

Chicken _____

Bioflavonoids (vitamin p, vitamin C) _____

Citrus mix _____

Berry mix _____

Fruit mix _____

Vinegar mix _____

Choline _____

Inositol _____

PABA _____

Biotin _____

Vitamin B1 _____

Vitamin B2 _____

Vitamin B3 _____

Vitamin B4 _____

Vitamin B5 _____

Vitamin B6 _____

Vitamin B12 _____

Vitamin B13 _____

Vitamin B15 _____

Vitamin B17 _____

Folic acid _____

Date sugar _____

Cane sugar _____

Beet sugar _____

Dextrose _____

Glucose _____

Fructose _____

Maltose _____

Brown sugar _____

Corn sugar _____

Rice sugar _____

Honey _____

Lactose _____

Maple sugar _____

Sorbitol _____

Aspartame _____

Saccharine _____

Sweet 'n' low _____

Equal _____

Red wine _____

White wine _____

MSG _____

Meat mix _____

Malathion _____

Pesticides _____

Plastics _____

Formaldehyde _____

Crude oil _____

Animal epithelial / Dander _____

Fabric mix _____

Insect mix _____

Grass mix _____

Pollen mix _____

Weed mix _____

Mold mix _____

Dust mix _____

Newspaper/ Ink _____

Mercury _____

Ttree mix _____

Flower mix _____

Freon _____

Radiation _____

Chemical mix _____

Virus mix _____

Bacteria mix _____

I.D. _____

Hormones _____

Smoking /Nicotine _____

Perfume Mix _____

Wood mix _____

Tetracycline _____

ITEMS TO TREAT TOGETHER

Certain items can be treated together if the patient is not very allergic to individual items. These items are:

1. Salt mix and chloride

2. Coffee mix, caffeine and chocolate mix

3. Nut mix 1 and nut mix 2

4. Spices 1 and spices 2

5. Yeast mix, yogurt, and whey

6. Fish mix and shell fish mix and vitamin A

7. Baking powder and baking soda

8. Newspaper and Newspaper ink

9. Animal epithelial/ Animal dander

10. Fabrics

11. Chemicals

DETAILED NAET TREATMENT GUIDE

1. EGG MIX.   (EGG YOLK, EGG WHITE, CHICKEN, TETRACYCLINE, FEATHERS).

YOU MAY NOT EAT OR TOUCH: egg white, egg yolk, chicken, tetracycline and all foods containing egg or chicken including crackers, cookies, soups, breads, mayonnaise, salad dressings, cakes, pastries, pies, pancakes, foods baked or fried in egg batter and thick sauces. Also avoid birds, feather pillows, comforters, vitamins and protein drinks made with egg, shampoos, conditioners and skin lotions with egg products.

YOU MAY EAT: brown or white rice, pasta without eggs, vegetables, fruits, milk products, oils, beef, pork, fish, coffee, juice, soft drinks, water and tea .

Date treated: _____   Cleared: _____

Combinations needed: Acid/.....Base/.....DNA/.....RNA/..... Heat/......Cold/...... (RNA+DNA)=N/ N+Acid/......N+Base/.....N+Heat/.... N+Cold/ .. N+Acid+Heat/ N+Base+Heat/... N+Acid+Cold/ N+Base+Cold/..... Organs (like Lung, heart, stomach, spleen, liver, gall bladder, pancreas, kidney, small intestines, urinary bladder, colon, uterus, prostate, brain, ovary, etc.) /.....Pituitrophin/..... Seratonin/.....Hormones/.....Emotional Blockage/...Emotional Blockage +Acid/... Emotional blockage + Base / ... Emotional blockage +RNA + DNA/Emotional blockage+HEAT/ ... Emotional Blockage +COLD/..... Emotional Blockage + RNA+DNA/ ... Emotional Blockage +RNA+DNA+ Acid/......Emotional Blockage + RNA + DNA +BASE /.... Emotional blockage + RNA + DNA + HEAT/.... Emotional blockage + RNA + DNA + cold/... Emotional blockage + Hormone/..... Emotional blockage + Serotonin/.....Eggs + Calcium/ Eggs + Vitamin C/ Eggs + B.Complex/ Eggs + Sugar/ ... Eggs + Calcium (Milk) + B. Complex (Flour) + Sugar+Spices (Cinnamon Cookies for example.)

One may find various reactive combinations like milk & cereal, breads, cookies, ice creams, various foods and drinks. After one completes the basic ingredients, one should combine everyday foods together like breakfast, lunch & dinner of Monday, or Tuesday etc. and treat them for reaction to the food combining. In following pages, followed by each allergen, the abbreviations of the combinations are given to save space in the book.

Symptoms Noted:_____

Notes:_____

_____

_____

2. CALCIUM MIX (Cal-Carbonate, Cal- Gluconate, Cal-ascorbate, Cow's milk, goat's milk, milk-casein, milk-albumin).

YOU MAY NOT EAT OR TOUCH: milk or milk products, uncooked vegetables, dark leafy vegetables like lettuce, cabbage, dandelion greens, Brussels sprouts, broccoli, sesame seeds, oats, navy beans, milk products, cheese, soybeans, almonds, dried beans, walnuts, sardines, salmon, peanuts, and sunflower seeds, calcium supplements.

YOU MAY EAT: cooked rice, pasta, cooked vegetables, cooked potato, corn, yams, cauliflower, sweet potato, red meat, and coffee and/or tea without milk. Drink calcium- free water. Any food without calcium derivatives

Date treated: _____   Cleared: _____

Combinations needed:..................... A/.....B/.....D/.....R/.....H/......C/.....N/..... N+A/...... N+B/
N+H/.....N+C/.....N+A+H/.....N+B+H/.....N+A+C/.....N+B+C/.....
EB/.....EB+A/.....EB+B/.....EB+N/.....EB+H/ ...EB+C/ ..... EB+N+A/....EB+N+B/.... EB+N+A+H/
.EB+N+B+H/....EB+N+A+C/...EB+N+B+C/.....

Symptoms
Noted:_____

Notes: _____

3. VITAMIN C MIX (Ascorbic acid, Oxalic acid, citrus mix, berry mix, fruit mix, vegetable mix, vinegar mix, chlorophyll, hesparin, rutin, bioflavanoids).

YOU MAY NOT EAT OR TOUCH: fresh fruits, vegetables, leafy vegetables, citrus fruits, dry fruits, juices, sauces, soft drinks, milk, artificial sweeteners, and vitamin C supplements.

YOU MAY EAT: cooked white or brown rice, pasta without sauce, boiled or poached eggs, baked or broiled chicken, fish, red meat, brown toast, deep fried food, french fries, salt, oils, and drink coffee and water. Any food that does not have vitamin C or its derivatives.

Date treated: _____   Cleared: _____
Combinations needed:.. A/.....B/.....D/.....R/.....H/......C/.....N/..... A/......N+B/...N+H/.....N+C/
N+A+H/...N+B+H/....N+A+C/...N+B+C/....EB/...EB+A/...EB+B/...EB+N/...EB+H/ ...EB+C/ ...
EB+N+A/...EB+N+B/... +N+A+H/....EB+N+B+H/.EB+N+A+C/...EB+N+B+C/.....

Symptoms
Noted:_____

Notes: _____

<u>4. B COMPLEX</u>. (B1, 2, 3, 4, 5, 6, 12, 13, 15, 17, paba, inositol, choline, biotin, folic acid).

YOU MAY NOT EAT OR TOUCH: whole grain products, fruits, vegetables, meats, dairy products, anything with B vitamins.

YOU MAY EAT: cooked white rice, cooked white pasta, cauliflower raw or cooked, well cooked or deep fried fish, salt, white sugar, black coffee, French fries, purified water while treating for any of the B vitamins. Rice should be washed well before cooking. Then, cook rice or pasta with lots of water and drain the water after cooking the rice (pasta) to remove the fortified vitamins. You may refer to the following individual B vitamins for more information.

<u>VITAMIN B1:</u> (thiamine, thiamine mononitrate, thiamine chloride, thiamine HCL)

AVOID: dried yeast, rice husks, whole wheat, oatmeal, peanuts, pork, most vegetables, bran, milk, brewer's yeast, wheat germ, wheat bran, rice polishings, most whole grain cereals, milk products, leafy green vegetables, meat, liver, nuts, legumes, and potatoes.

YOU MAY EAT: white rice, white flour pasta, raw or cooked cauliflower, cooked or deep fried fish, french fries, white sugar, purified water, and black coffee.

<u>VITAMIN B2:</u> (riboflavin, Vitamin G)

AVOID: milk, cheese, whole grains, brewer's yeast, wheat germ, almonds, sunflower seeds, liver, cooked leafy vegetables, kidney, raw or broiled fish and eggs.

YOU MAY EAT: white rice, white flour pasta, raw or cooked cauliflower, cooked or deep fried fish, french fries, white sugar, purified water, and black coffee.

<u>VITAMIN B3:</u> (niacin, nicotinic acid, niacinamide)

AVOID : lean meat, raw or broiled fish, eggs, roasted peanuts, brewer's yeast, wheat germ, rice bran, rice polishings, nuts, sunflower seeds, whole wheat products, brown rice, green vegetables, liver, white meat of poultry, avocado, dates, figs, and prunes.

YOU MAY EAT: white rice, white flour pasta, raw or cooked cauliflower, cooked or deep fried fish, French fries, white sugar, water, and black coffee.

<u>Vitamin B4 :</u> (Adenine)

AVOID: whole grains, leafy vegetables, and nuts.

YOU MAY EAT: white rice, white flour pasta, raw or cooked cauliflower, cooked or deep fried fish, French fries, white sugar, purified water, and black coffee.

<u>Vitamin B5:</u> (pantothenic acid, calcium pantothenate)

AVOID: Brewers yeast, wheat germ, wheat bran, royal jelly, whole grain breads and cereals, green vegetables, peas, dried beans, nuts, crude molasses, raisins, cantaloupe, red meat, liver, kidney, heart, egg yolk, and chicken.

YOU MAY EAT: white rice, white flour pasta, raw or cooked cauliflower, cooked or deep fried fish, French fries, white sugar, purified water, and black coffee.

Vitamin B6: (pyridoxine, pyridoxine HCL)

AVOID: brewer's yeast, bananas, avocado, wheat germ, wheat bran, soybeans,

milk, green leafy vegetables, cabbage, molasses, green peppers, legumes, cantaloupe, egg yolk, organ meats, kidney, heart, liver, and beef.

YOU MAY EAT: white rice, white flour pasta, raw or cooked cauliflower, cooked or deep fried fish, French fries, white sugar, purified water, and black coffee.

Vitamin B12: (cobalamin, cyanocobalamin)

AVOID: milk, eggs, aged cheese, yogurt, bee pollen, flower pollen, meat, liver, pork and kidney.

YOU MAY EAT: white rice, white flour pasta, raw or cooked cauliflower, cooked or deep fried fish, French fries, white sugar, purified water, and black coffee.

Vitamin B13: (orotic acid)

AVOID: milk-whey (the liquid portion of soured or curdled milk) and root vegetables.

YOU MAY EAT: white rice, white flour pasta, raw or cooked cauliflower, cooked or deep fried fish, French fries, white sugar, purified water, and black coffee.

Vitamin B15: (pangamic acid, calcium pangamate)

AVOID: whole grains, nuts, whole brown rice, brewer's yeast, pumpkin seeds and sesame seeds.

YOU MAY EAT: white rice, white flour pasta, raw or cooked cauliflower, cooked or deep fried fish, French fries, white sugar, purified water, and black coffee.

Vitamin B17: (nitrilosides, amygdalin, laetrile)

AVOID: Most whole seeds of fruits and many grains and vegetables, raspberries, cranberries, blackberries, blueberries, mung beans, lima beans, flaxseeds, whole kernels of apricots, apples, cherries, peaches, plums and nectarines.

YOU MAY EAT: white rice, white flour pasta, raw or cooked cauliflower, cooked or deep fried fish, French fries, white sugar, purified water, and black coffee.

BIOTIN: (Vitamin H, coenzyme R)

AVOID: brewer's yeast, unpolished rice, soybeans, liver, kidney, milk, molasses, nuts, fruit, beef and yolks.

YOU MAY EAT: white rice, white flour pasta, raw or cooked cauliflower, cooked or deep fried fish, French fries, white sugar, purified water, and black coffee.

CHOLINE:

AVOID: brewer's yeast, wheat germ, egg yolk, liver, green leafy vegetables, legumes, peas, beans, brain, heart and lecithin.

YOU MAY EAT: white rice, white flour pasta, raw or cooked cauliflower, cooked or deep fried fish, French fries, white sugar, purified water, and black coffee.

INOSITOL:

AVOID: brewer's yeast, wheat germ, lecithin, unprocessed whole grains, nuts, milk, citrus fruits, liver, dried lima beans, beef, brains, heart, raisins, cantaloupe, unrefined molasses, peanuts and cabbage.

YOU MAY EAT: white rice, white flour pasta, raw or cooked cauliflower, cooked or deep fried fish, French fries, white sugar, purified water, and black coffee.

FOLIC ACID: (Vitamin B 9, Pteroylglutamic Acid, Folate Folacin).

AVOID: dark green leafy vegetables, broccoli, asparagus, lima beans, Irish potatoes, brewer's yeast, wheat germ, mushrooms, nuts, liver, carrots, tortilla, yeast, egg yolk, cantaloupe, apricots, pumpkins, avocados, beans, whole wheat and dark rye flour.

YOU MAY EAT: white rice, white flour pasta, raw or cooked cauliflower, cooked or deep fried fish, French fries, white sugar, purified water, and black coffee.

PABA: (Para Amino Benzoic Acid, Vitamin BX)

AVOID: brewer's yeast, whole grain products, milk, eggs, yogurt, wheat germ, molasses, liver, kidney, whole grains, rice and bran.

YOU MAY EAT: white rice, white flour pasta, raw or cooked cauliflower, cooked or deep fried fish, French fries, white sugar, purified water, and black coffee.

Date treated: _____ Cleared: _____

Combinations needed:............................. A/.....B/.....D/.....R/.....H/......C/.....N/..... N+A/......N+B/ N+H/...N+C/.....N+A+H/.....N+B+H/.....N+A+C/.....N+B+C/.....EB/.....EB+A/.....EB+B/.....EB+N/ EB+H/ ...EB+C/ ..... EB+N+A/....EB+N+B/.... B+N+A+H/EB+N+B+H/....EB+N+A+C/...EB+N+B+C/

Symptoms Noted:_____

Notes:_____

5. SUGAR MIX: (cane sugar, beet sugar, brown sugar, corn sugar, rice sugar, maple sugar, molasses, honey, fruit sugar, sucrose, glucose, dextrose, maltose, lactose, date sugar, grape sugar).

YOU MAY NOT EAT: anything with any of the above sugars, sauces, drinks with sugar. Do not use powdered spices in pre-packed containers, tooth paste and mouth washing liquids.

YOU MAY EAT: white rice, pasta, vegetables, vegetable oils, meats, eggs, chicken, water, coffee, tea without milk.

Date treated: _____ Cleared: _____

Combinations needed:............................. A/.....B/.....D/.....R/.....H/......C/.....N/.....
N+A/......N+B/.....N+H/.....N+C/.....N+A+H/.....N+B+H/.....N+A+C/.....N+B+C/.
EB/.....EB+A/.....EB+B/.....EB+N/.....EB+H/ ...EB+C/ ..... EB+N+A/....EB+N+B/....
EB+N+A+H/....EB+N+B+H/....EB+N+A+C/...EB+N+B+C/.....

Symptoms Noted:_____

Notes:_____
_____

6. IRON MIX (ferrous sulfate, ferrous gluconate, beef, pork, lamb, gelatin).

YOU MAY NOT EAT OR TOUCH: apricots, peaches, banana, black molasses, dates, prunes, raisins, brewer's yeast, whole grain cereals, turnip greens, broccoli, Brussels sprout, spinach, beet tops, alfalfa, beets, sunflower seeds, walnuts, sesame seeds, whole rye, dry beans, lentils, kelp, egg yolk, liver, red meat, pork liver, beef, organ meats like kidney, heart and liver, farina, raw clams, oysters, nuts, asparagus, coffee, chocolate and iron supplements.

YOU MAY EAT: white rice without iron fortification, sour dough bread without iron, cauliflower, potato, chicken, light green vegetables, water and orange juice.

Date treated: _____ Cleared: _____

Combinations needed:............................. A/.....B/.....D/.....R/.....H/......C/.....N/..... N+A/......N+B/
N+H/.....N+C/.....N+A+H/.....N+B+H/.....N+A+C/.....N+B+C/.....
EB/.....EB+A/.....EB+B/.....EB+N/.....EB+H/ ...EB+C/ ..... EB+N+A/....EB+N+B/.... EB+N+A+H/
EB+N+B+H/....EB+N+A+C/...EB+N+B+C/.....

Symptoms
Noted:_____

Notes:_____

7. VITAMIN A MIX: FISH, SHELL FISH MIX

(beta carotene, vitamin A, fish, shellfish sources).

YOU MAY NOT USE OR TOUCH: yellow fruits, yellow vegetables, green fruits, green vegetables, green peppers, fish or fish products, milk products and corn products.

YOU MAY USE: steamed rice, pasta, potato, cauliflower, red apples, chicken, water and coffee.

Date treated: _____ Cleared: _____

Combinations needed:.................................. A/.....B/.....D/.....R/.....H/......C/.....N/..... N+A/......N+B/ H/.....N+C/.....N+A+H/.....N+B+H/.....N+A+C/.....N+B+C/.....

EB/.....EB+A/.....EB+B/.....EB+N/.....EB+H/ ...EB+C/ ..... EB+N+A/....EB+N+B/.... EB+N+A+H/ EB+N+B+H/....EB+N+A+C/...EB+N+B+C/.....

Symptoms
Noted:_____

Notes: _____

_____

8. MINERAL MIX (trace minerals like antimony, barium, boron, beryllium, bromide, caesium, chlorine, chromium, cobalt, copper, europium, fluorine, gallium, germanium, gold, iodine, lithium, manganese, molybdenum, nickel, palladium, rubidium, samarium, scandium, silver, strontium, thallium, thorium, tin, titanium, tungsten, uranium, zinc, zirconium, chromium, lead, magnesium, manganese, phosphorus, potassium, selenium, sulfur, vanadium, mercury).

YOU MAY NOT USE OR TOUCH: metals, tap water, mineral water, root vegetables like onion, potato, carrots and turnips. Wear gloves while touching metal surfaces. Metal buttons on clothes, shoes, hand bags, wedding rings or religious rings etc. can be covered with masking tape. Use plastic and glass utensils to cook and eat. Use a pair of gloves during 25 hour period to avoid touching metals.

YOU MAY USE: distilled water for washing and showering, steamed rice, vegetables, fruits, meats, eggs, milk, coffee and tea.

Date treated:_____ Cleared: _____

Combinations needed:.................................. A/.....B/.....D/.....R/.....H/......C/.....N/..... N+A/......N+B/ N+H/.....N+C/.....N+A+H/.....N+B+H/.....N+A+C/.....N+B+C/.....

EB/.....EB+A/.....EB+B/.....EB+N/.....EB+H/ ...EB+C/ ..... EB+N+A/....EB+N+B/... EB+N+A+H/ EB+N+B+H/....EB+N+A+C/...EB+N+B+C/.....

Symptoms Noted:_____

Notes:_____

9. SALT MIX, CHLORIDES: (sea salt, table salt, rock salt, sodium and chloride).

YOU MAY NOT USE OR TOUCH: kelp, celery, romaine lettuce, watermelon, sea food, processed foods with salts, fast foods, table salts, fish, shell fish, carrots, beets, artichoke, dried beef, brains, kidney, cured meats, bacon, ham, coffee, watercress, sea weed, oats, avocado, Swiss chard, tomatoes, cabbage, cucumber, asparagus, pineapple, tap water, and prepared , canned or frozen foods.

YOU MAY USE: distilled water to drink and bathe, steamed rice, fresh vegetables and fruits not listed above, chicken, meats and sugars.

Date treated: _____ Cleared: _____

Combinations needed:............................. A/.....B/.....D/.....R/.....H/......C/..... N/...... N+A/.....
N+B/.....N+H/.....N+C/.....N+A+H/.....N+B+H/.....N+A+C/.....N+B+C/.....EB/.....EB+A/.....
EB+B/.....EB+N/.....EB+H/ ...EB+C/ ..... EB+N+A/....EB+N+B/ .... B+N+A+H/....
EB+N+B+H/....EB+N+A+C/...EB+N+B+C/.....

Symptoms Noted:
_____

Notes:_____

10. CORN MIX: (blue corn, yellow corn, white corn, cornstarch, cornsilk, corn oat, corn syrup).

AVOID: corn starch and any food prepared with corn starch and oil such as sauces, syrups, corn syrups, soft drinks, carbonated drinks, breads, creams. Also avoid shampoos, tooth paste, baking soda, baking powder, and deodorants.

YOU MAY USE: steamed vegetables, steamed rice, broccoli, baked chicken, and meats. You may drink water, tea and/or coffee without cream or sugar.

Date treated: _____ Cleared: _____

Combinations needed:............................. A/.....B/.....D/.....R/.....H/......C/.....N/....
N+A/......N+B/.....N+H/.....N+C/.....N+A+H/.....N+B+H/.....N+A+C/.....N+B+C/....
EB/.....EB+A/.....EB+B/.....EB+N/.....EB+H/ ...EB+C/ ..... EB+N+A/....EB+N+B/EB+N+A+H/
B+N+B+H/....EB+N+A+C/...EB+N+B+C/.....

Symptoms Noted:_____

Notes:_____

11. GRAIN MIX: (wheat, corn, rice, oats, rye, millet, barley).

YOU MAY NOT USE: grains and items made from above grains.

YOU MAY EAT: vegetables, fruits, meats, milk and drink water.

Date treated: _____ Cleared: _____

Combinations needed:....................................... A/.....B/.....D/.....R/.....H/......C/ EB/.....EB+A/
EB+B/.....EB+N/.....EB+H/ ...EB+C/ ..... EB+N+A/....EB+N+B/.... EB+N+A+H/....EB+N+B+H/
EB+N+A+C/...EB+N+B+C/.....

Symptoms
Noted:_____

Notes:_____

_____

12. YEAST MIX: (Baker's Yeast, Brewer's Yeast, Tortula Yeast, candida albicans).

AVOID: Brewer's yeast, bakers yeast, and any foods containing these items
including baked goods, sugars, fruits, soy sauce, and alcoholic beverages.

YOU MAY EAT vegetables, meat, chicken and fish.

Date treated: _____ Cleared: _____

Combinations needed:.. A/...B/...D/...R/...H/...C/...N/...N+A/...N+B/...N+H/...N+C/... N+A+H/
N+B+H/...N+A+C/...N+B+C/...EB/...EB+A/...EB+B/...EB+N/...
EB+H/...EB+C/...EB+N+A/...EB+N+B/...EB+N+A+H/...EB+N+B+H/.... EB+N+A+C/...
EB+N+B+C/.....

Symptoms Noted:_____

Notes:_____

_____

13. ARTIFICIAL SWEETENERS: (Equal, Nutrasweet, Aspartame, Sorbitol, Sweet And Low Saccharine, Twin).

AVOID: items with the above artificial sugars, like soft drinks, sweet relish, pickles, sauces, cookies, tooth paste, mouthwash, etc.

YOU MAY EAT: anything without artificial sweeteners. Use freshly prepared items only.

Date treated: _____ Cleared: _____

Combinations needed:.............................. A/.....B/.....D/.....R/.....H/......C/.....

N/.....N+A/......N+B/.....N+H/.....N+C/.....N+A+H/.....N+B+H/.....N+A+C/.....

N+B+C/..... EB/.....EB+A/.....EB+B/.....EB+N/.....EB+H/ ...EB+C/ .....

EB+N+A/....EB+N+B/....EB+N+A+H/....EB+N+B+H/....EB+N+A+C/...

EB+N+B+C/.....

Symptoms
Noted:_____

Notes:_____

14. COFFEE MIX: Coffee, chocolate mix, caffeine, tea, tannic acid, cocoa, cocoa butter, carob.

YOU MAY NOT USE OR SMELL: Coffee, tea, caffeinated drinks, leather goods, tannic acids.

YOU MAY EAT: anything that has no coffee, caffeine or chocolate.

Date treated: _____ Cleared: _____

Combinations needed:.. A/...B/...D/...R/...H/...C/...N/...N+A/...N+B/... N+H/...N+C/... N+A+H/ N+B+H/...N+A+C/... N+B+C/... EB/...EB+A/...EB+B/... EB+N/...EB+H/... EB+C/ ... EB+N+A/... EB+N+B/...EB+N+A+H/...EB+N+B+H/... EB+N+A+C/... EB+N+B+C/...

Symptoms
Noted:_____

Notes:_____

15. CHOCOLATE MIX: Chocolate mix, caffeine, cocoa, cocoa butter, carob.

YOU MAY NOT USE OR SMELL: chocolate and all foods containing chocolate: ice cream.

YOU MAY EAT: anything that has no chocolate.

Date treated: _____ Cleared: _____

Combinations needed:.. A/...B/...D/...R/...H/...C/...N/...N+A/...N+B/... N+H/...N+C/... N+A+H/...N+B+H/...N+A+C/... N+B+C/... EB/...EB+A/...EB+B/... EB+N/...EB+H/... EB+C/ ... EB+N+A/...EB+N+B/...EB+N+A+H/...EB+N+B+H/... EB+N+A+C/... EB+N+B+C/...

Symptoms
Noted:_____

Notes:_____
_____

16. CAFFEINE: Coffee, caffeine, tea, tannic acid, carob.

YOU MAY NOT USE OR SMELL: Coffee, tea, caffeinated drinks, leather goods, tannic acids.

YOU MAY EAT: anything that has no coffee, caffeine.

Date treated: _____ Cleared: _____

Combinations needed:.. A/...B/...D/...R/...H/...C/...N/...N+A/...N+B/... N+H/...N+C/... N+A+H/...N+B+H/...N+A+C/... N+B+C/... EB/...EB+A/...EB+B/... EB+N/...EB+H/... EB+C/ ... EB+N+A/...EB+N+B/...EB+N+A+H/...EB+N+B+H/... EB+N+A+C/... EB+N+B+C/...

Symptoms
Noted:_____

Notes:_____

17. NUT MIX 1 (peanuts, black walnut, English walnut).

YOU MAY NOT EAT OR TOUCH: peanuts, walnuts, black walnuts, and English walnuts or anything made from these nuts or their oils.

YOU MAY EAT: any foods that do not contain the nuts listed above including their oils and butters.

Date treated: _____ Cleared: _____

Combinations needed:.. A/...B/...D/...R/...H/...C/...N/...N+A/...N+B/...N+H/...
N+C/.....N+A+H/.....N+B+H/.....N+A+C/...N+B+C/...EB/...EB+A/...
EB+B/...EB+N/... EB+H/ ...EB+C/ ... EB+N+A/...EB+N+B/...EB+N+A+H/... EB+N+B+H/
EB+N+A+C/...EB+N+B+C/.....

Symptoms
Noted:_____
Notes:_____

18. NUT MIX 2 (cashew, almonds, pecan, Brazil nut, hazelnut, macadamia, sunflower seeds).

YOU MAY NOT EAT OR TOUCH: any of the above mentioned nuts or oils.
YOU MAY EAT: any foods that do not contain the nuts listed above including their oils and butters.

Date treated:_____ Cleared: _____
Combinations needed:.. A/...B/...D/...R/...H/...C/...N/...N+A/....N+B/...
N+H/.....N+C/.....N+A+H/.....N+B+H/.....N+A+C/.....N+B+C/.....
EB/.....EB+A/.....EB+B/.....EB+N/.....EB+H/ ...EB+C/ ..... EB+N+A/....EB+N+B/....
EB+N+A+H/....EB+N+B+H/....EB+N+A+C/...EB+N+B+C/.....

Symptoms Noted:_____
Notes:_____

19. SPICE MIX 1 (ginger, cardamom, cinnamon, cloves, nutmeg, garlic, cumin, fennel, coriander, turmeric, saffron, mint).

AVOID: above listed spices in any form. These spices and their oils are encountered in candies, chewing gums, tooth paste, massage oils, aroma therapy ingredients and toiletries.

YOU MAY USE: all foods, and products without these items.

Date treated: _____ Cleared: _____

combinations needed:.. A/...B/...D/...R/...H/....C/...N/...N+A/...N+B/...N+H/...N+C/...N+A+H/ ...N+B+H/...N+A+C/...N+B+C/...EB/...EB+A/...EB+B/...EB+N/...EB+H/ ...EB+C/... EB+N+A/ ...EB+N+B/...EB+N+A+H/...

EB+N+B+H/...EB+N+A+C/...EB+N+B+C/...

Symptoms Noted: _____

Notes:_____

20. SPICE MIX 2 (peppers, red pepper, black pepper, green pepper, jalapino, banana peppers, anise seed, basil, bay leaf, caraway seed, chervil, cream of tartar, dill, fenugreek, horseradish, mace, MSG, mustard, onion, oregano, paprika, poppy seed, parsley, rosemary, sage, sumac, and vinegar).

AVOID: any of the above spices.

YOU MAY USE: all foods and food products without the above listed spices.

Date treated: _____Cleared: _____

Combnations needed:... A/...B/...D/...R/...H/...C/...N/...N+A/....N+B/...N+H/...

N+C/...N+A+H/...N+B+H/...N+A+C/...N+B+C/...EB/...EB+A/...EB+B/...

EB+N/.....EB+H/ ...EB+C/ ..... EB+N+A/....EB+N+B/...EB+N+A+H/...

EB+N+B+H/...EB+N+A+C/...EB+N+B+C/....

Symptoms Noted: _____

Notes:_____

21. ANIMAL FAT: (butter, lard, chicken fat, beef fat, lamb fat, fish oil).

YOU MAY NOT USE OR TOUCH: butter, lard, meats, fish and fish oils, skin lotions with lanolin or animal fat, food fried in animal fat, refried beans, chili beans, corn chips fried in lard etc.

YOU MAY USE: anything other than the above including vegetable oils.

Date treated: _____ Cleared: _____

Combinations needed:... A/...B/...D/...R/...H/....C/...N/...N+A/...N+B/...N+H/...
N+C/...N+A+H/...N+B+H/...N+A+C/...N+B+C/...EB/...EB+A/...EB+B/...
EB+N/...EB+H/ ...EB+C/ ... EB+N+A/...EB+N+B/...EB+N+A+H/...
EB+N+B+H/...EB+N+A+C/...EB+N+B+C/...

Symptoms Noted:_____

Notes:_____

22. VEGETABLE FATS: (Corn oil, canola oil, peanut oil, linseed oil, sun flower oil, palm oil, flax seed oil, coconut oil).

YOU MAY NOT USE: vegetable oils, foods containing vegetable oils like breads, crackers, cookies, sauces, drinks, and skin lotions, makeup items, shampoo, conditioner etc.

YOU MAY USE: steamed vegetables, steamed rice, meats, eggs, chicken, butter and animal fats.

Date treated: _____ Cleared: _____

Combinations needed:..... A/...B/...D/...R/...H/....C/...N/...N+A/....N+B/...
N+H/...N+C/...N+A+H/...N+B+H/...N+A+C/...N+B+C/...EB/...EB+A/...
EB+B/...EB+N/...EB+H/ ...EB+C/ .... EB+N+A/...EB+N+B/...
EB+N+A+H/...EB+N+B+H/...EB+N+A+C/... EB+N+B+C/...

Symptoms Noted:_____

Notes:_____

23. AMINO ACIDS 1: (essential amino acids: Lysine, methionine, leucine, threonine, Valine, thryptophan, isoleucine, and phenylalanine).

YOU MAY NOT EAT OR TOUCH: any type of food that contains proteins, and protein products that are used for external application.

YOU MAY EAT: steamed white rice, lettuce and drink water.

Date treated:_____ Cleared: _____

Combinations needed:.. A/...B/...D/...R/...H/...C/...N/...N+A/...N+B/...N+H/...N+C/... N+A+H/ N+B+H/...N+A+C/...N+B+C/...EB/...EB+A/...EB+B/...EB+N/... EB+H/...EB+C/...EB+N+A/...EB+N+B/...EB+N+A+H/...EB+N+B+H/.... EB+N+A+C/... EB+N+B+C/

Symptoms Noted:_____

Notes:_____

24. AMINO ACIDS 11: (non essential amino acids: alanine, arginine, aspartic acid, carnitine, citrulline, cysteine, glutathione, glutamic acid, glycine, histidine, ornithine, proline, serine, taurine, tyrosine).

YOU MAY NOT EAT OR TOUCH: any type of food that contains proteins, and protein products that are used for external application.

YOU MAY EAT: steamed white rice, lettuce and drink water.

Date treated:_____ Cleared: _____

Combinations needed:.. A/...B/...D/...R/...H/...C/...N/...N+A/...N+B/...N+H/...N+C/... N+A+H/ N+B+H/...N+A+C/...N+B+C/...EB/...EB+A/...EB+B/...EB+N/... EB+H/...EB+C/...EB+N+A/...EB+N+B/...EB+N+A+H/...EB+N+B+H/.... EB+N+A+C/... EB+N+B+C/

Symptoms Noted:_____

Notes:_____

25. FISH MIX: (Cod, Halibut, Salmon, Tuna, Shark).

YOU MAY NOT EAT OR SMELL tuna, salmon, halibut, cod, their oils, and glues on the stamps, envelops, and anything else made from fish source.

YOU MAY EAT any food that does not contain the fish or fish oils listed above.

Date treated: _____   Cleared: _____

Combinations needed:.. A/...B/...D/...R/...H/...C/...N/...N+A/...N+B/...N+H/...
N+C/...N+A+H/...N+B+H/...N+A+C/...N+B+C/...EB/...EB+A/...EB+B/...
EB+N/...EB+H/ ...EB+C/ ... EB+N+A/...EB+N+B/...EB+N+A+H/...
EB+N+B+H/...EB+N+A+C/...EB+N+B+C/...

Symptoms Noted:_____

Notes:_____

_____

26. SHELLFISH MIX: (Shrimp, lobster, abalone, cray, crab, clams).

YOU MAY NOT EAT OR SMELL any fish or fish products.

YOU MAY EAT any food that does not contain fish products.

Date treated: _____   Cleared: _____

Combinations needed:.. A/...B/...D/...R/...H/...C/...N/...N+A/...N+B/...N+H/...
N+C/...N+A+H/...N+B+H/...N+A+C/...N+B+C/...EB/...EB+A/...EB+B/...
EB+N/...EB+H/ ...EB+C/ ... EB+N+A/...EB+N+B/...EB+N+A+H/...
EB+N+B+H/...EB+N+A+C/...EB+N+B+C/...

Symptoms Noted:_____

Notes:_____

27. WHEY:

AVOID: Cottage cheese, all yogurts and items made with whey like crackers, french breads, yogurt or cheese.

YOU MAY EAT rice, vegetables, fruits, chicken, egg, turkey, beef, pork, beans, and lamb.

Treated: _____ Cleared: _____

Combinations needed:.. A/...B/...D/...R/...H/...C/...N/...N+A/...N+B/...N+H/...N+C/... N+A+H/...N+B+H/...N+A+C/...N+B+C/...EB/...EB+A/...EB+B/...EB+N/... EB+H/...EB+C/...EB+N+A/...EB+N+B/...EB+N+A+H/...EB+N+B+H/.... EB+N+A+C/... EB+N+B+C/.....

Symptoms Noted:_____

Notes:_____

_____

28. YOGURT

AVOID: cottage cheese, all yogurts, and items made with whey, yogurt or cheese.

YOU MAY EAT rice, vegetables, fruits, poultry, and meat.

Date treated: _____ Cleared: _____

Combinations needed:.. A/...B/...D/...R/...H/...C/...N/...N+A/...N+B/...N+H/...N+C/... N+A+H/
N+B+H/...N+A+C/...N+B+C/...EB/...EB+A/...EB+B/...EB+N/... EB+H/...EB+C/...EB+N+A/
EB+N+B/...EB+N+A+H/...EB+N+B+H/.... EB+N+A+C/... EB+N+B+C/.....

Symptoms Noted:_____

Notes:_____

_____

29. DRIED BEANS MIX : (Pinto beans, lima beans, lentils, peas, garbanzo beans, black beans, red beans, black eye peas, mung beans, navy beans).

AVOID: above listed beans, their oils or products.

YOU MAY EAT anything other than beans or bean products (rice, pasta,

vegetables, meats, eggs etc.).

Date treated: _____ Cleared. _____

Combinations needed:.. A/...B/...D/...R/...H/...C/...N/...N+A/...N+B/...N+H/...N+C/... N+A+H/ ...N+B+H/...N+A+C/...N+B+C/...EB/...EB+A/...EB+B/...EB+N/...

EB+H/...EB+C/...EB+N+A/...EB+N+B/...EB+N+A+H/...EB+N+B+H/.... EB+N+A+C/... EB+N+B+C/

Symptoms Noted:_____

Notes:_____

_____

30. TURKEY: (turkey, serotonin).

AVOID: Turkey in any form, milk products, tryptophane, vitamin B1, B3 and B6 and all the products with these vitamins (vitamin B1, B3, B6, tryptophane are the precursors of serotonin).

YOU MAY EAT any food that does not contain the above listed items.

Date treated: _____ Cleared: _____

Combinations needed:.. A/...B/...D/...R/...H/...C/...N/...N+A/...N+B/...N+H/...N+C/... N+A+H/ .N+B+H/...N+A+C/...N+B+C/...EB/...EB+A/...EB+B/...EB+N/...

EB+H/...EB+C/...EB+N+A/...EB+N+B/...EB+N+A+H/...EB+N+B+H/.... EB+N+A+C/... EB+N+B+C/.....

SymptomsNoted:_____

Notes_____

31. WHITEN-ALL

AVOID: Uncooked vegetables, fresh fruits, frozen vegetables, canned foods, potato salads, fruit salads made at the restaurant, or pre packed by catering companies, french fries, baked potato, any other potato prepared by caterers, sauces, dips, etc.

YOU MAY EAT Cooked vegetables, pasta, rice, meats, chicken and eggs.

Date treated: _____ Cleared: _____

Combinations needed:.. A/...B/...D/...R/...H/...C/...N/...N+A/...N+B/...N+H/...N+C/... N+A+H/ N+B+H/...N+A+C/...N+B+C/...EB/...EB+A/...EB+B/...EB+N/...

EB+H/...EB+C/...EB+N+A/...EB+N+B/...EB+N+A+H/...EB+N+B+H/.... EB+N+A+C/... EB+N+B+C/

Symptoms Noted:_____

Notes:_____

32. FLUORIDE

AVOID: Fluoridated water, gelatin, sunflower seeds, milk, cheese, carrots, garlic, almonds, green leafy vegetables and fish. Do not bathe in or drink fluoridated water. Do not eat products prepared with sunflower oil.

YOU MAY USE OR EAT fruits, poultry, meat, potato, cauliflower, white rice, and yellow vegetables. If you are also treating for water you may drink fresh fruit juices, and distilled water.

Date treated: _____ Cleared: _____

Combinations needed:.. A/...B/...D/...R/...H/...C/...N/...N+A/...N+B/...N+H/...N+C/... N+A+H/ N+B+H/... N+A+C/...N+B+C/...EB/...EB+A/...EB+B/...EB+N/...EB+H/...EB+C/...EB+N+A/... EB+N+B/...EB+N+A+H/...EB+N+B+H/.... EB+N+A+C/... EB+N+B+C/.....

Symptoms Noted:_____

Notes:_____

33. GELATIN

AVOID: Apple skin, pectin, hard skin of other fruits, okra, gelatin from chicken, meat, gelatin capsules, Jell-O, gelatin- added puddings, sticky candy, cosmetics, facial masks, and other makeup products.

YOU MAY USE the things that do not contain gelatin.

Date treated: _____ Cleared: _____

Combinations needed:.. A/...B/...D/...R/...H/...C/...N/...N+A/...N+B/...N+H/...N+C/...
N+A+H/...N+B+H/...N+A+C/...N+B+C/...EB/...EB+A/...EB+B/...EB+N/...EB+H/...
EB+C/...EB+N+A/...EB+N+B/...EB+N+A+H/...EB+N+B+H/.... EB+N+A+C/... EB+N+B+C/.....

Symptoms Noted:_____

Notes:_____

34. ALCOHOL: (beer, red wine, white wine, rubbing alcohol, cooking wine, champagne, tequila and vodka.)

AVOID : All alcoholic beverages, vanilla ice cream, foods cooked with wine, sugar and starchy foods, fruits, hair sprays, medicine with alcohols like cough syrups, shampoos, hair products, cosmetics and makeup products and rubbing alcohols.

YOU MAY USE Things not listed above. May eat vegetables, meats, fish, eggs and chicken.

Date treated: _____ Cleared: _____

Combinations needed:.. A/...B/...D/...R/...H/...C/...N/...N+A/...N+B/...N+H/...N+C/... N+A+H/
N+B+H/...N+A+C/...N+B+C/...EB/...EB+A/...EB+B/...EB+N/...EB+H/...EB+C/...
EB+N+A/...EB+N+B/...EB+N+A+H/...EB+N+B+H/.... EB+N+A+C/... EB+N+B+C/.....

Symptoms Noted: _____

Notes: _____

35. BAKING POWDER/ BAKING SODA

AVOID: Baking powder, baking soda, and foods, medications and tooth pastes, deodorants, antiperspirants, talcum powders, soaps, detergents, cotton crotches of female underpants, containing baking soda.

YOU MAY EAT OR USE any foods which do not contain the items listed above including fresh fruits, vegetables, fats, meat and chicken.

Date treated: _____ Cleared: _____

Symptoms Noted:_____

Notes:_____

36. GUM MIX: Acacia, Karaya gum, Xanthine gum, Black gum, Sweet gum and chewing gum.

AVOID : Soft drinks, glues, chewing gum, cream cheese, and carbonated drinks. Please read the labels on the food containers if you are buying from the market.

YOU MAY USE things not containing gums. You may eat rice, pasta, vegetables, fruits without skins, meats, eggs and chicken.

Date treated: _____ Cleared: _____

Combinations needed:............ A/.....B/.....D/.....R/.....H/......C/.....N/.....N+A/......N+B/....N+H/... N+C/ N+A+H/.....N+B+H/.....N+A+C/.....N+B+C/....EB/.....EB+A/.....EB+B/.....EB+N/.....EB+H/ ...EB+C/ EB+N+A/....EB+N+B/....EB+N+A+H/....EB+N+B+H/.... EB+N+A+C/...EB+N+B+C/

Symptoms Noted:_____

Notes:_____

37. VEGETABLE MIX

AVOID: Avoid all vegetables and items made with vegetables. Add all available local vegetables while treating with this sample.

YOU MAY EAT OR USE any foods which do not contain the items listed above.

Date treated: _____ Cleared: _____

Symptoms Noted:_____

Notes:_____

<u>38. VITAMIN D:</u> (Ergosterol, Viosterol, Calciferol, Cholecalciferol or Cholecalciferol, Ergocalciferol, Sunshine Vitamin).

AVOID: Fish liver oil, egg yolks, milk, butter, sprouted seeds, mushrooms, sunflower seeds and sunflower oil.

YOU MAY EAT any foods not listed above including fruits, vegetables, poultry and meat.

Date treated: _____   Cleared: _____

Combinations needed:.. A/...B/...D/...R/...H/...C/...N/...N+A/...N+B/...N+H/...N+C/... N+A+H/...N+B+H/...N+A+C/...N+B+C/...EB/...EB+A/...EB+B/...EB+N/...EB+H/...EB+C/...EB+N+A/...EB+N+B/...EB+N+A+H/...EB+N+B+H/.... EB+N+A+C/... EB+N+B+C/.....

Symptoms noted:_____

Notes:_____

<u>39. VITAMIN E</u>
(Tocopherol, d-Alpha Tocopherol, or Tocopheryl, D1-Alpha Tocopherol, or Tocopheryl, Mixed Tocopherols).

AVOID: Wheat germ, soybeans, vegetable oils, broccoli, brussel sprouts, leafy greens, spinach, enriched flour, whole wheat, whole grain cereals, eggs, unrefined cold pressed crude vegetable oils, wheat germ and soybean oils, whole, raw or sprouted seeds, nuts and grains.

YOU MAY EAT fresh fruit, carrots, potatoes, poultry and meat.

Date treated: _____   Cleared: _____

Combinations needed:.. A/...B/...D/...R/...H/...C/...N/...N+A/...N+B/...N+H/...N+C/... N+A+H/
N+B+H/...N+A+C/...N+B+C/...EB/...EB+A/...EB+B/...EB+N/.. EB+H/...EB+C/...EB+N+A/
EB+N+B/...EB+N+A+H/...EB+N+B+H/.... EB+N+A+C/... EB+N+B+C/.....

Symptoms Noted:_____

Notes:_____

40. VITAMIN K: (phytomenadione, phytonadione, phylloquinone, menadione).

AVOID : Kelp, alfalfa and other green plants, soybean oils, egg yolks, cow's milk, liver, yogurt, safflower and soybean oils, fish liver oils, cabbage, Brussels sprouts and green leafy vegetable.

YOU MAY EAT : Fruit, rice, potato, poultry and meat.

Date treated:_____ Cleared :_____

Combinations needed:.. A/...B/...D/...R/...H/...C/...N/...N+A/...N+B/...N+H/...N+C/... N+A+H/...N+B+H/...N+A+C/...N+B+C/...EB/...EB+A/...EB+B/...EB+N/... EB+H/...EB+C/...EB+N+A/...EB+N+B/...EB+N+A+H/...EB+N+B+H/.... EB+N+A+C/... EB+N+B+C/.....

Symptoms Noted: _____

Notes:_____

41. VITAMIN F: (Unsaturated fatty acids-linoleic, gamma-linoleic and arachinoidic factors).

AVOID: Vegetable oils, wheat germ oils, linseed oils, sunflower oils, safflower oils, soybean oils, peanuts and peanut oils, flax seeds, evening primrose oils, all nuts and breast milk.

YOU MAY EAT anything that is not in the above list.

Date treated:_____ Cleared:_____

Combinations needed:.. A/...B/...D/...R/...H/...C/...N/...N+A/...N+B/...N+H/...N+C/...
N+A+H/...N+B+H/...N+A+C/...N+B+C/...EB/...EB+A/...EB+B/...EB+N/...EB+H/...EB+C/...
EB+N+A/...EB+N+B/...EB+N+A+H/...EB+N+B+H/.... EB+N+A+C/...EB+N+B+C/.....

Symptoms Noted:_____

Notes:_____

42. <u>VITAMIN P:</u> (Bioflavanoids, citrus bioflavonoids, hesperidin, rutin). This is very essential for venous and capillary integrity.

AVOID: Rose hips, buckwheat, citrus fruit pulp, green peppers, grapes, apricot, strawberries, black currants, cherries, prunes, white skin and segment part of citrus fruit, oranges, grapefruit, lemons and black berries.

YOU MAY EAT things not in the above list.

Date treated: _____   Cleared: _____

Combinations needed:.. A/...B/...D/...R/...H/...C/...N/...N+A/...N+B/...N+H/...N+C/...
N+A+H/...N+B+H/...N+A+C/...N+B+C/...EB/...EB+A/...EB+B/...EB+N/... EB+H/...
EB+C/...EB+N+A/...EB+N+B/...EB+N+A+H/...EB+N+B+H/.... EB+N+A+C/... EB+N+B+C/

Symptoms Noted: _____

Notes:_____

43. <u>VITAMIN T:</u> (sesame seed factor).

AVOID: sesame seeds, egg yolks, vegetable oils.

YOU MAY EAT anything other than in the above list.

Date treated:_____   Cleared: _____

Combinations needed:.. A/...B/...D/...R/...H/...C/...N/...N+A/...N+B/...N+H/...N+C/... N+A+H/
N+B+H/...N+A+C/...N+B+C/...EB/...EB+A/...EB+B/...EB+N/... EB+H/...EB+C/...EB+N+A/
EB+N+B/...EB+N+A+H/...EB+N+B+H/.... EB+N+A+C/... EB+N+B+C/.

Symptoms Noted: _____

Notes:_____

44. RNA/DNA

AVOID : All type of proteins.

YOU MAY EAT white rice and lettuce.

Date treated: _____ Cleared: _____

Combinations needed:.. A/...B/...D/...R/...H/...C/...N/...N+A/...N+B/...N+H/...N+C/...
N+A+H/...N+B+H/...N+A+C/...N+B+C/...EB/...EB+A/...EB+B/...EB+N/...EB+H/..
EB+C/...EB+N+A/...EB+N+B/...EB+N+A+H/...EB+N+B+H/.... EB+N+A+C/... EB+N+B+C/.....

Symptoms Noted:_____
Notes:_____
_____

45. STOMACH ACIDS

AVOID : Sugar, starches, fruits, grains, meats, other acid forming foods, coffee.

YOU MAY EAT raw and steamed vegetables, cooked dried beans, eggs, oils, clarified butter, and milk.

Date treated:_____ Cleared : _____

Combinations needed:.. A/...B/...D/...R/...H/...C/...N/...N+A/...N+B/...N+H/...N+C/... N+A+H/...
N+B+H/...N+A+C/...N+B+C/...EB/...EB+A/...EB+B/...EB+N/...EB+H/...EB+C/...EB+N+A/...
EB+N+B/...EB+N+A+H/...EB+N+B+H/.... EB+N+A+C/... EB+N+B+C/.....

Symptoms Noted:_____
Notes:_____

46. BASE: (Digestive juices and enzymes from intestinal tracts).

AVOID : Raw and cooked vegetables, beans , eggs, and milk.

YOU MAY EAT sugars, starches, breads and meats.

Date treated:_____ Cleared:_____

Combinations needed:.. A/...B/...D/...R/...H/...C/...N/...N+A/...N+B/...N+H/...N+C/... N+A+H/...
N+B+H/...N+A+C/...N+B+C/...EB/...EB+A/...EB+B/...EB+N/... EB+H/...EB+C/...EB+N+A/..
EB+N+B/...EB+N+A+H/...EB+N+B+H/.... EB+N+A+C/... EB+N+B+C/.....

Symptoms Noted:_____

Notes:_____

47. Pituitrophin (PT) (Check in case of hormonal imbalance, dizzy spells, headaches at the back of the neck).

Avoid meats and eggs

YOU MAY EAT fresh vegetables, rice, pasta, fish and water.

48. SEROTONIN(One of the brain enzymes responsible for relaxation. Check in cases with insomnia, attention deficit hyperactive disorders, depression, manic disorders, autism and frequent respiratory tract infections, frequent bronchitis, and flu's):

Avoid turky, asparagus, avocado, cocoa, pineapple, plum, tomato, yeast, milk, milk products, B1, B3, B6 and tryptophane.

YOU MAY EAT fresh vegetables and fruits not on the list, rice, pasta, fish and water.

49. FOOD COLORING (Check in cases with ADD, Autism, restless leg syndrome, sweating of the palms).

AVOID colored foods, pre mixed powdered spices, frozen vegetables, sauces, candies, chewing gums, soft drinks, ice creams, lipstick, crayons, coloring books, etc.

YOU MAY EAT fresh vegetables, rice, pasta, eggs, chicken, milk and water.

Date treated:_____ Cleared: _____

Combinations needed:.. A/...B/...D/...R/...H/...C/...N/...N+A/...N+B/...N+H/...N+C/... N+A+H/ N+B+H/...N+A+C/...N+B+C/...EB/...EB+A/...EB+B/...EB+N/... EB+H/...EB+C/...EB+N+A/ EB+N+B/...EB+N+A+H/...EB+N+B+H/.... EB+N+A+C/... EB+N+B+C/.....

Symptoms Noted:_____

Notes:_____

50. FOOD ADDITIVES: (Sodium nitrate, sodium phosphates, calcium sulfates, calcium phosphates). (Check in cases with seizure disorders, hyperactivity, migraines, muscle aches, arthritis, anorexia, anorexia nervosa).

AVOID : Hot dogs, sausages, pre-packed meats, soups, crackers, certain cookies (read labels), salad dressings, sauces etc.

YOU MAY EAT : Fresh vegetables, freshly cooked grains, eggs, chicken and milk.

Date treated:_____ Cleared: _____

Combinations needed:.. A/...B/...D/...R/...H/...C/...N/...N+A/...N+B/...N+H/...N+C/... N+A+H/ N+B+H/...N+A+C/...N+B+C/...EB/...EB+A/...EB+B/...EB+N/... EB+H/...EB+C/...EB+N+A/ EB+N+B/...EB+N+A+H/...EB+N+B+H/.... EB+N+A+C/... EB+N+B+C/.....

Symptoms Noted:_____

Notes:_____

These following items are included in the mineral mix. After you clear the mineral mix, must check these individually.

51. CHROMIUM (Check in case of diabetes).

AVOID: Whole grains, wheat germ, corn oil, brewers yeast, mushrooms, meat,

Liver, sugar, shellfish, clams, chicken.

YOU MAY EAT : White rice and pasta, cauliflower, potato, fruits, table salt, drink water.

Date treated:_____ Cleared: _____

Combinations needed:.. A/...B/...D/...R/...H/...C/...N/...N+A/...N+B/...N+H/...N+C/...

N+A+H/...N+B+H/...N+A+C/...N+B+C/...EB/...EB+A/...EB+B/...EB+N/... EB+H/...

EB+C/...EB+N+A/...EB+N+B/...EB+N+A+H/...EB+N+B+H/.... EB+N+A+C/... EB+N+B+C/.....

52. COBALT (Check in case of anemia).

AVOID : Green leafy vegetables, meat, liver, kidney, figs, buckwheat, oyster, clams, milk.

YOU MAY EAT: white rice and pasta, cauliflower, potato, fresh fruits, non iodized salt, drink water.

Date treated:_____ Cleared: _____

Combinations needed:.. A/...B/...D/...R/...H/...C/...N/...N+A/...N+B/...N+H/...N+C/... N+A+H/

.N+B+H/...N+A+C/...N+B+C/...EB/...EB+A/...EB+B/...EB+N/... EB+H/...EB+C/...

EB+N+A/...EB+N+B/...EB+N+A+H/...EB+N+B+H/.... EB+N+A+C/... EB+N+B+C/.....

Symptoms Noted:_____

Notes:_____

53. COPPER (Check in case of arthritis and anemia).

AVOID almonds, green beans, peas, green leafy vegetables, whole grains, prunes, raisins, liver, dried beans, whole wheat, beef liver, calf liver, shrimp, seafood.

YOU MAY EAT white rice and pasta, cauliflower, potato, fresh fruits, non iodized salt, drink water.

Date treated:_____ Cleared: _____

Combinations needed:.. A/...B/...D/...R/...H/...C/...N/...N+A/...N+B/...N+H/...N+C/...
N+A+H/...N+B+H/...N+A+C/...N+B+C/...EB/...EB+A/...EB+B/...EB+N/... EB+H/...EB+C/
.EB+N+A/...EB+N+B/...EB+N+A+H/...EB+N+B+H/.... EB+N+A+C/... EB+N+B+C/.....

Symptoms Noted:_____

Notes:_____

54 .GERMANIUM (Check in cases with arthritis and fatigue).

AVOID all whole grains and sprouts including breads.

YOU MAY EAT fruit, vegetables, vegetable oils, dairy, poultry and meats.

Date treated:_____ Cleared: _____

Combinations needed:.. A/...B/...D/...R/...H/...C/...N/...N+A/...N+B/...N+H/...N+C/... N+A+H/
...N+B+H/...N+A+C/...N+B+C/...EB/...EB+A/...EB+B/...EB+N/... EB+H/...EB+C/...EB+N+A/
...EB+N+B/...EB+N+A+H/...EB+N+B+H/.... EB+N+A+C/... EB+N+B+C/.....

Symptoms Noted:_____

Notes:_____

55. Gold (Check in cases with arthritis, lupus, fibromyalgia)..

Avoid gold and all yellow metal in any form

YOU MAY EAT fruit, vegetables, vegetable oils, dairy, poultry and meats.

Date treated:_____ Cleared: _____

Combinations needed:.. A/...B/...D/...R/...H/...C/...N/...N+A/...N+B/...N+H/...N+C/... N+A+H/
...N+B+H/...N+A+C/...N+B+C/...EB/...EB+A/...EB+B/...EB+N/... EB+H/...EB+C/...EB+N+A/
...EB+N+B/...EB+N+A+H/...EB+N+B+H/.... EB+N+A+C/... EB+N+B+C/.....

Symptoms Noted:_____

Notes:_____

56. IODINE (Check in cases with chronic fatigue, thyroid imbalance, hives, fish and shellfish allergy).

AVOID kelp, seafood, iodized salt, onions.

YOU MAY EAT rice and pasta, cauliflower, potato, fruits, non iodized salt, drink water.

Date treated:_____ Cleared: _____

Combinations needed:.. A/...B/...D/...R/...H/...C/...N/...N+A/...N+B/...N+H/...N+C/... N+A+H/...N+B+H/...N+A+C/...N+B+C/...EB/...EB+A/...EB+B/...EB+N/... EB+H/...EB+C/...EB+N+A/...EB+N+B/...EB+N+A+H/...EB+N+B+H/.... EB+N+A+C/... EB+N+B+C/.....

Symptoms Noted:_____

Notes:_____

57. LEAD (Check in cases with brain fog, heaviness in the brain and limbs, allergy to tap water),

AVOID tap water, lead pencil.

YOU MAY EAT anything that is not cooked in tap water.

Date treated:_____ Cleared: _____

Combinations needed:.. A/...B/...D/...R/...H/...C/...N/...N+A/...N+B/...N+H/...N+C/... N+A+H/...N+B+H/...N+A+C/...N+B+C/...EB/...EB+A/...EB+B/...EB+N/... EB+H/...EB+C/...EB+N+A/...EB+N+B/...EB+N+A+H/...EB+N+B+H/.... EB+N+A+C/... EB+N+B+C/.....

Symptoms Noted:_____

Notes:_____

58. MAGNESIUM (Check in cases with chronic constipation, eczema, asthma, breathing difficulty, liver toxicity, water retention anywhere in the body).

AVOID nuts, soybeans, raw and cooked green leafy vegetables, almonds, whole grains, sunflower seeds, brown rice, sesame seeds.

YOU MAY EAT white rice, potato, cauliflower, eggs, chicken, meats, milk and fruits.

Date treated:_____ Cleared: _____

Combinations needed:.. A/...B/...D/...R/...H/...C/...N/...N+A/...N+B/...N+H/...N+C/... N+A+H/... N+B+H/..EB+H/ ...EB+C/ ..... +N+A/....EB+N+B/... EB+N+A+H/.... EB+N+B+H/.... EB+N+A+C/ EB+N+B+C/.....

Symptoms Noted:_____

Notes:_____

59. Manganese (Retention of water in the body, weight gain in the waist area, clinical depression, mood swings, and if you think you are alone in this world and no one loves you).

AVOID whole grains, seeds, nuts, legumes, dairy products, egg yolks, fish, corn dried fruits, poultry and meat.

YOU MAY EAT steamed white rice, potato, cauliflower, fresh fruit, fresh vegetable and vegetable oil.

Date treated:_____ Cleared: _____

Combinations needed:.. A/...B/...D/...R/...H/...C/...N/...N+A/...N+B/...N+H/...N+C/... N+A+H/... N+B+H/...N+A+C/...N+B+C/...EB/...EB+A/...EB+B/...EB+N/... EB+H/...EB+C/...EB+N+A/EB+N+B/ ...EB+N+A+H/...EB+N+B+H/.... EB+N+A+C/... EB+N+B+C/.....

Symptoms Noted:_____

Notes:_____

60. MOLYBDENUM

AVOID whole grains, brown rice, brewers yeast, legumes, buck wheat, millet, dark green and leafy vegetables.

YOU MAY EAT steamed white rice, potato, cauliflower, fresh fruits, non-iodized salt and water.

Date treated:_____ Cleared: _____

Combinations needed:.. A/...B/...D/...R/...H/...C/...N/...N+A/...N+B/...N+H/...N+C/... N+A+H/... N+B+H/...N+A+C/...N+B+C/...EB/...EB+A/...EB+B/...EB+N/... EB+H/...EB+C/...EB+N+A/EB+N+B/ ...EB+N+A+H/...EB+N+B+H/.... EB+N+A+C/... EB+N+B+C/.....

Symptoms Noted:_____

Notes:_____

61. PHOSPHORUS (Check in cases with General body ache, chronic fatigue, fibromyalgia, pain in the joints).

AVOID whole grains, seeds, nuts, legumes, dairy products, egg yolks, fish, corn dried fruits, poultry and meat.

YOU MAY EAT steamed white rice, potato, cauliflower, fresh fruit, fresh vegetable and vegetable oil.

Date treated:_____ Cleared: _____

Combinations needed:.. A/...B/...D/...R/...H/...C/...N/...N+A/...N+B/...N+H/...N+C/... N+A+H/
...N+B+H/...N+A+C/...N+B+C/...EB/...EB+A/...EB+B/...EB+N/... EB+H/...EB+C/...EB+N+A/
...EB+N+B/...EB+N+A+H/...EB+N+B+H/.... EB+N+A+C/... EB+N+B+C/.....

Symptoms Noted:_____

Notes:_____

62. POTASSIUM (Check in cases with fatigue, heart irregularities, brain fog,)

AVOID all vegetables, oranges, bananas, cantaloupe, tomatoes, mint leaves, water cress, potatoes, whole grains, seeds, nuts, and cream of tartar.

YOU MAY EAT white rice and pasta, cauliflower, chicken, meat, eggs.

Date treated:_____ Cleared: _____

Combinations needed:.. A/...B/...D/...R/...H/...C/...N/...N+A/...N+B/...N+H/...N+C/... N+A+H/...
N+B+H/...N+A+C/...N+B+C/...EB/...EB+A/...EB+B/...EB+N/... EB+H/...EB+C/...EB+N+A/
EB+N+B/...EB+N+A+H/...EB+N+B+H/.... EB+N+A+C/... EB+N+B+C/.....

Symptoms Noted:_____

Notes:_____

63. SELENIUM (Check in cases with liver toxicity, heart irregularities, shortness of brath).

AVOID brewers yeast, wheat germ, kelp, sea water, sea salt, garlic, mushrooms, sea food, milk, eggs, whole grains, beef, beans, bran, onions, tomato, broccoli.

YOU MAY EAT white rice and pasta, cauliflower, potato, chicken, fruits, table salt, drink water.

Date treated:_____ Cleared: _____

Combinations needed:.. A/...B/...D/...R/...H/...C/...N/...N+A/...N+B/...N+H/...N+C/... N+A+H/.. N+B+H/...N+A+C/...N+B+C/...EB/...EB+A/...EB+B/...EB+N/... EB+H/...EB+C/...EB+N+A/ EB+N+B/...EB+N+A+H/...EB+N+B+H/.... EB+N+A+C/... EB+N+B+C/.....

Symptoms Noted:_____

Notes:_____

64. SILVER (Check in cases with Mercury toxicity, night sweats, brain fog).
(silver jewelry, coins, utensils, anything made from silver, teeth fillings, any medicine containing silver).

AVOID all all of the above silver products.

YOU MAY EAT vegetables, meats, eggs, beans.

Date treated:_____ Cleared: _____

Combinations needed:.. A/...B/...D/...R/...H/...C/...N/...N+A/...N+B/...N+H/...N+C/... N+A+H/... N+B+H/...N+A+C/...N+B+C/...EB/...EB+A/...EB+B/...EB+N/... EB+H/...EB+C/...EB+N+A/...EB+N+B/...EB+N+A+H/...EB+N+B+H/.... EB+N+A+C/... EB+N+B+C/

Symptoms Noted:_____

Notes:_____

65. .SULFUR (Check in cases with eczema, toxic colon).

AVOID radish, turnip, onion, celery, string beans, watercress, soybean, fish, meat, dried beans, eggs, cabbage.

YOU MAY EAT: white rice and pasta, cauliflower, potato, fruits, non iodized salt, drink water.

Date treated:_____ Cleared:_____

Combinations needed:.. A/...B/...D/...R/...H/...C/...N/...N+A/...N+B/...N+H/...N+C/... N+A+H/
N+B+H/...N+A+C/...N+B+C/...EB/...EB+A/...EB+B/...EB+N/... EB+H/...EB+C/...EB+N+A/
EB+N+B/...EB+N+A+H/...EB+N+B+H/.... EB+N+A+C/... EB+N+B+C/.....

Symptoms Noted:_____

Notes:_____

66. VANADIUM (Check in cases with heavy metal toxicity).
AVOID fish, seafood.

YOU MAY EAT everything that is not seafood.

Date treated:_____ Cleared: _____

Combinations needed:...................................... A/.....B/.....D/.....R/.....H/......C/.....N/
N+A/......N+B/.....N+H/.....N+C/.....N+A+H/.....N+B+H/.....N+A+C/.....N+B+C/.....EB/.....EB+A/.....
EB+B/.....EB+N/.....EB+H/ ...EB+C/ ..... EB+N+A/....EB+N+B/....EB+N+A+H/.... EB+N+B+H/
EB+N+A+C/...EB+N+B+C/.....

Symptoms Noted:_____

Notes:_____

67. ZINC(Check in cases with immune disorders, frequent flu like symptoms, eczema, hormonal disorders, enlarged prostate, infertility in both sexes, low libido).

AVOID wheat bran, wheat germ, seeds, dried beans, peas, onions, mushrooms, brewers yeast, milk, eggs, oysters, herring, brown rice, fish, lamp, beef, pork, green leafy vegetables, mustard.

YOU MAY EAT white rice and pasta, cauliflower, potato, chicken, table salt, drink water.

Date treated:_____ Cleared: _____

Combinations needed:.. A/...B/...D/...R/...H/...C/...N/...N+A/...N+B/...N+H/...N+C/... N+A+H/ N+B+H/...N+A+C/...N+B+C/...EB/...EB+A/...EB+B/...EB+N/...EB+H/...EB+C/...EB+N+A/ EB+N+B/...EB+N+A+H/...EB+N+B+H/.... EB+N+A+C/... EB+N+B+C/

Symptoms Noted:_____

Notes:_____

68. SOYBEAN MIX (Check in cases with hormonal disorders, lumps in the breast, fibrocystic breast, uterine fibroids).

AVOID all soy products including soy oil, soy milk, soy curd or tofu.

YOU MAY EAT everything without soybean product.

Date treated:_____ Cleared: _____

Combinations needed:.. A/...B/...D/...R/...H/...C/...N/...N+A/...N+B/...N+H/...N+C/... N+A+H/ N+B+H/...N+A+C/...N+B+C/...EB/...EB+A/...EB+B/...EB+N/... EB+H/...EB+C/...EB+N+A/ EB+N+B/ EB+N+A+H/...EB+N+B+H/.... EB+N+A+C/... EB+N+B+C/.....

Symptoms Noted:_____

Notes:_____

69. LECITHIN (Check in cases with brain fog, poor memory, arteriosclerosis, pain in the calf muscles,)

AVOID lecithin products, including cookies, candy bars, vitamins with lecithin, soy lecithin etc.

YOU MAY EAT white rice, cauliflower, potato, water.

Date treated: _____ Cleared:_____

Combinations needed:.. A/...B/...D/...R/...H/...C/...N/...N+A/...N+B/...N+H/...N+C/...
N+A+H/...N+B+H/...N+A+C/...N+B+C/...EB/...EB+A/...EB+B/...EB+N/...EB+H/...EB+C/...
EB+N+A/...EB+N+B/...EB+N+A+H/...EB+N+B+H/.... EB+N+A+C/... EB+N+B+C/.....

Symptoms Noted:_____

Notes:_____

70. MILK MIX: (Cow's milk, goat's milk, breast milk).

AVOID all milk products.

YOU MAY EAT everything without milk.

Date treated: _____ Cleared: _____

Combinations needed:.. A/...B/...D/...R/...H/...C/...N/...N+A/...N+B/...N+H/...N+C/...
N+A+H/...N+B+H/...N+A+C/...N+B+C/...EB/...EB+A/...EB+B/...EB+N/...EB+H/...EB+C/...
EB+N+A/...EB+N+B/...EB+N+A+H/...EB+N+B+H/.... EB+N+A+C/... EB+N+B+C/.....

Symptoms Noted:_____

Notes:_____

71. CHEESE MIX: (American, cheddar, jack, parmesan, mozzarella , cottage).

AVOID all products made from cheese.

YOU MAY EAT everything other than cheese.

Date treated: _____ Cleared: _____

Combinations needed:.. A/...B/...D/...R/...H/...C/...N/...N+A/...N+B/...N+H/...N+C/...
N+A+H/...N+B+H/...N+A+C/...N+B+C/...EB/...EB+A/...EB+B/...EB+N/... B+H/...EB+C/...
EB+N+A/...EB+N+B/...EB+N+A+H/...EB+N+B+H/.... EB+N+A+C/... EB+N+B+C/

Symptoms Noted:_____

Notes:_____

_____

72. TOMATO MIX: (green, yellow, red tomato).

AVOID tomatoes of all kinds, and the products made from tomato.

YOU MAY EAT everything without tomato or it's product.

Date treated: _____ Cleared: _____

Combinations needed:.. A/...B/...D/...R/...H/...C/...N/...N+A/...N+B/...N+H/...N+C/... N+A+H/...N+B+H/
...N+A+C/...N+B+C/...EB/...EB+A/...EB+B/...EB+N/... EB+H/...EB+C/...EB+N+A/...EB+N+B/
...EB+N+A+H/...EB+N+B+H/.... EB+N+A+C/... EB+N+B+C/

Symptoms Noted:_____

Notes:_____

73. ONION MIX: (brown, red, white, green). One of the nightshade vegetables, others:pepper, potato, tomato and egg plant).

AVOID onions and the products made from onions.

YOU MAY EAT everything except onions.

Date treated: _____   Cleared:_____

Combinations needed:.. A/...B/...D/...R/...H/...C/...N/...N+A/...N+B/...N+H/...N+C/...
N+A+H/...N+B+H/...N+A+C/...N+B+C/...EB/...EB+A/...EB+B/...EB+N/...
EB+H/...EB+C/...EB+N+A/...EB+N+B/...EB+N+A+H/...EB+N+B+H/.... EB+N+A+C/... EB+N+B+C/

74. PEPPER MIX: (red, green, black, yellow, Mexican, Italian, Indian peppers).

AVOID all peppers and anything made from peppers.

YOU MAY EAT anything other peppers.

Date treated: _____   Cleared: _____

Combinations needed:.. A/...B/...D/...R/...H/...C/...N/...N+A/...N+B/...N+H/...N+C/...
N+A+H/...N+B+H/...N+A+C/...N+B+C/...EB/...EB+A/...EB+B/...EB+N/... EB+H/..
.EB+C/...EB+N+A/...EB+N+B/...EB+N+A+H/...EB+N+B+H/.... EB+N+A+C/... EB+N+B+C/.....

Symptoms Noted:_____

Notes:_____

75. POTATO MIX: (russet, white, red, sweet, yam. Potato contains solanin).

AVOID all type of potatoes and the products made from potato.

YOU MAY EAT anything that does not have potato.

Date treated: _____   Cleared: _____

Combinations needed:.. A/...B/...D/...R/...H/...C/...N/...N+A/...N+B/...N+H/...N+C/...
N+A+H/...N+B+H/...N+A+C/...N+B+C/...EB/...EB+A/...EB+B/...EB+N/...
EB+H/...EB+C/...EB+N+A/...EB+N+B/...EB+N+A+H/...EB+N+B+H/.... EB+N+A+C/... EB+N+B+C/

Symptoms Noted:_____

Notes: _____

_____

76. WHEAT MIX: (red, buck wheat, white, gluten, coumarin).

AVOID all wheat products.

YOU MAY EAT everything other than wheat products.

Date treated:_____ Cleared: _____

Combinations needed:.. A/...B/...D/...R/...H/...C/...N/...N+A/...N+B/...N+H/...N+C/...
N+A+H/...N+B+H/...N+A+C/...N+B+C/...EB/...EB+A/...EB+B/...EB+N/...EB+H/...EB+C/...EB+N+A/
...EB+N+B/...EB+N+A+H/...EB+N+B+H/.... EB+N+A+C/... EB+N+B+C/

Symptoms Noted: _____

Notes:_____

77. CUCUMBER MIX: (green, pickled).

AVOID: Cucumber and pickles and products made from cucumber like soaps, salad dressings, face creams etc.

YOU MAY EAT anything that doesn't have cucumber.

Date treated:_____ Cleared: _____

Combinations needed:.. A/...B/...D/...R/...H/...C/...N/...N+A/...N+B/...N+H/...N+C/... N+A+H/...
N+B+H/...N+A+C/...N+B+C/...EB/...EB+A/...EB+B/...EB+N/... EB+H/...EB+C/...EB+N+A/...
EB+N+B/...EB+N+A+H/...EB+N+B+H/.... EB+N+A+C/... EB+N+B+C/.....

Symptoms Noted:_____

Notes: _____

78. MELON MIX: (Crenshaw, water, cantaloupe, honey dew, pumpkin).

AVOID all types of melons.

YOU MAY EAT everything else other than melon.

Date treated:_____ Cleared:_____

Combinations needed:.. A/...B/...D/...R/...H/...C/...N/...N+A/...N+B/...N+H/...N+C/... N+A+H/... N+B+H/..N+A+C/..N+B+C/..EB/..EB+A/..EB+B/..EB+N/..EB+H/..EB+C/..EB+N+A/ EB+N+B/...EB+N+A+H/...EB+N+B+H/.... EB+N+A+C/... EB+N+B+C/

Symptoms Noted:_____

Notes:_____
_____

79. MODIFIED STARCH: (refined starches from Potato, corn, arrow root, rice, all purpose flour).

AVOID all starch products, refined grain products, vitamins, certain prescription drugs (read labels), table salt, thick sauces.

YOU MAY EAT vegetables, meats, eggs, beans.

Date treated:_____ Cleared: _____

Combinations needed:.. A/...B/...D/...R/...H/...C/...N/...N+A/...N+B/...N+H/...N+C/... N+A+H/... N+B+H/...N+A+C/...N+B+C/...EB/...EB+A/...EB+B/...EB+N/... EB+H/...EB+C/...EB+N+A/...EB+N+B/...EB+N+A+H/...EB+N+B+H/.... EB+N+A+C/... EB+N+B+C/

Symptoms Noted:_____

Notes:_____
_____

OTHER ALLERGENS / ENVIRONMENTAL ALLERGENS

Egg White / Egg Yolk
 Chicken / Tetracycline   Please look up under Egg Mix

Bioflavonoids / Citrus Mix
 Berry Mix / Fruit Mix   Please look up under Vitamin C Mix
Vinegar Mix

Choline / Inositol / PABA
 Biotin / Vitamin B1
Vitamin B2 / Vitamin B3   Please look up under B Complex
 Vitamin B4
Vitamin B5 / Vitamin B6
 Vitamin B12 / Vitamin B13
 Vitamin B15 / Vitamin B17
Folic Acid

Date Sugar/ Cane Sugar
 Beet Sugar/ Dextrose
 Glucose/ Fructose   Please look up under Sugar Mix
 Maltose /Brown Sugar
Rice Sugar/ Corn Sugar
 Honey/ Lactose/ Maple Sugar.

SORBITOL/ ASPARTAME   Please look up under Artificia Sweetners
SACCHARINE
 SWEET 'N' LOW/ EQUAL

WHITE WINE/ RED WINE

AVOID red or white wine or any food prepared with wine. Avoid sulfites and red and green grapes.

You may eat anything else.

Date treated:_____   Cleared: _____

Combinations needed:.. A/...B/...D/...R/...H/...C/...N/...N+A/...N+B/...N+H/...N+C/... N+A+H/...
N+B+H/...N+A+C/...N+B+C/...EB/...EB+A/...EB+B/...EB+N/... EB+H/...EB+C/...
EB+N+A/   EB+N+B/   EB+N+A+H/   EB+N+B+H/.... EB+N+A+C/... EB+N+B+C/.....

Symptoms Noted:_____

Notes:_____

MSG

AVOID eating anything prepared with MSG or Accent.

You may eat anything else.

Date treated:_____   Cleared: _____

Combinations needed:.. A/...B/...D/...R/...H/...C/...N/...N+A/...N+B/...N+H/...N+C/... N+A+H/...
N+B+H/...N+A+C/...N+B+C/...EB/...EB+A/...EB+B/...EB+N/... EB+H/...EB+C/..
EB+N+A/...EB+N+B/...EB+N+A+H/...EB+N+B+H/.... EB+N+A+C/... EB+N+B+C/.....

Symptoms Noted:_____

Notes:_____

PARASITE MIX: (Pin worm, tape worm, hook worm, amoeba, giardia, protozoa)

AVOID eating anything uncooked. Drink boiled water.

Date treated:_____   Cleared: _____

Combinations needed:.. A/...B/...D/...R/...H/...C/...N/...N+A/...N+B/...N+H/...N+C/... N+A+H/...
N+B+H/...N+A+C/...N+B+C/...EB/...EB+A/...EB+B/...EB+N/... EB+H/...EB+C/...EB+N+A/...
EB+N+B/...EB+N+A+H/...EB+N+B+H/.... EB+N+A+C/... EB+N+B+C/.....

Symptoms Noted:_____

Notes:_____

PESTICIDES/.MALATHAION

AVOID fresh vegetables, fruits, meats, insecticides, new mattress, malathion sprays, ant bates, and house, grass, weeds, lawns, trees that have been sprayed for pesticides.

YOU MAY EAT cooked grains, vegetables and fruits.

Date treated: _____ Cleared: _____

Combinations needed:.. A/...B/...D/...R/...H/...C/...N/...N+A/...N+B/...N+H/...N+C/... N+A+H/... N+B+H/...N+A+C/...N+B+C/...EB/...EB+A/...EB+B/...EB+N/...EB+H/...EB+C/...EB+N+A/... EB+N+B/...EB+N+A+H/...EB+N+B+H/.... EB+N+A+C/... EB+N+B+C/.....

Symptoms Noted:_____

Notes: _____

_____

PLASTICS

AVOID all plastic and crude oil products including computer key boards, tele-phones, pens, vinyl chairs, containers, book covers, toothbrush, hair brush etc.

Date treated:_____ Cleared: _____ _____

Combinations needed:.. A/...B/...D/...R/...H/...C/...N/...N+A/...N+B/...N+H/...N+C/... N+A+H/... N+B+H/...N+A+C/...N+B+C/...EB/...EB+A/...EB+B/...EB+N/...EB+H/...EB+C/...EB+N+A/... EB+N+B/...EB+N+A+H/...EB+N+B+H/.... EB+N+A+C/... EB+N+B+C/.....

Symptoms Noted:_____

Notes:_____

FORMALDEHYDE

AVOID new buildings, new clothes, newspaper, liquid paper, pressed woods, paints, paint thinners, fumes, perfumes, certain ice creams. Wear a mask and use a pair of gloves. Remove name tags from the clothes or tape them with masking tape.

Wear mask and gloves if necessary.

Date treated:_____ Cleared: _____

Combinations needed:.. A/...B/...D/...R/...H/...C/...N/...N+A/...N+B/...N+H/...N+C/... N+A+H/... N+B+H/...N+A+C/...N+B+C/...EB/...EB+A/...EB+B/...EB+N/... EB+H/...EB+C/...EB+N+A/... EB+N+B/...EB+N+A+H/...EB+N+B+H/.... EB+N+A+C/... EB+N+B+C/.....

Symptoms Noted:_____

Notes:_____

CRUDE OIL

AVOID: Gasoline, plastc products, latex products. Wear gloves and mask if necessary.

Date treated:_____ Cleared: _____

Combinations needed:.. A/...B/...D/...R/...H/...C/...N/...N+A/...N+B/...N+H/...N+C/... N+A+H/... N+B+H/...N+A+C/...N+B+C/...EB/...EB+A/...EB+B/...EB+N/...EB+H/...EB+C/...EB+N+A/... EB+N+B/...EB+N+A+H/...EB+N+B+H/.... EB+N+A+C/... EB+N+B+C/.....

Symptoms Noted:_____

Notes:_____

_____

ANIMAL EPITHELIAL/ANIMAL DANDER.

AVOID contact with the animals, their saliva, hair, danders, any other products made from animals or used by the animals. If you have a pet, make arrangements to stay away from him/her for 25 hours.

Date treated:_____

Cleared: _____

Combinations needed:.. A/...B/...D/...R/...H/...C/...N/...N+A/...N+B/...N+H/...N+C/... N+A+H/... N+B+H/...N+A+C/...N+B+C/...EB/...EB+A/...EB+B/...EB+N/...EB+H/...EB+C/...EB+N+A/.. .EB+N+B/...EB+N+A+H/...EB+N+B+H/.... EB+N+A+C/... EB+N+B+C/.....

Symptoms Noted:_____

Notes:_____

_____

FABRIC MIX

Try to treat one kind of fabric first, like cotton or polyester etc. Then wear the allergy-cleared item while treating for the fabric mix.

AVOID contact with the fabric that is being treated.

Date treated:_____   Cleared: _____

Combinations needed:.. A/...B/...D/...R/...H/...C/...N/...N+A/...N+B/...N+H/...N+C/... N+A+H/ ...N+B+H/ ...N+A+C/...N+B+C/...EB/...EB+A/...EB+B/...EB+N/...

INSECT MIX: (Bee, ant, spider, flea).

AVOID touching or going near any insects.

Date treated:_____

Cleared: _____

Combinations needed:.. A/...B/...D/...R/...H/...C/...N/...N+A/...N+B/...N+H/...N+C/... N+A+H/ ...N+B+H/...N+A+C/...N+B+C/...EB/...EB+A/...EB+B/...EB+N/...

EB+H/...EB+C/...EB+N+A/...EB+N+B/...EB+N+A+H/...EB+N+B+H/.... EB+N+A+C/... EB+N+B+C/

Symptoms Noted:_____

Notes:_____

GRASS MIX

AVOID going out doors. Wear shoes and socks while walking outside.

Date treated:_____ Cleared: _____

Combinations needed:.. A/...B/...D/...R/...H/...C/...N/...N+A/...N+B/...N+H/...N+C/... N+A+H/...N+B+H/...N+A+C/...N+B+C/...EB/...EB+A/...EB+B/...EB+N/...

EB+H/...EB+C/...EB+N+A/...EB+N+B/...EB+N+A+H/...EB+N+B+H/.... EB+N+A+C/... EB+N+B+C/

Symptoms Noted:_____

Notes:_____

POLLEN MIX

AVOID going out doors. Wear a mask.

Date treated: _____ Cleared: _____

Combinations needed:.. A/...B/...D/...R/...H/...C/...N/...N+A/...N+B/...N+H/...N+C/... N+A+H/...
N+B+H/...N+A+C/...N+B+C/...EB/...EB+A/...EB+B/...EB+N/... EB+H/...EB+C/...EB+N+A/...
EB+N+B/...EB+N+A+H/...EB+N+B+H/.... EB+N+A+C/... EB+N+B+C/

Symptoms Noted:_____

Notes:_____

WEED MIX

AVOID going out doors. Wear a mask.

Date treated: _____ Cleared: _____

Combinations needed:.. A/...B/...D/...R/...H/...C/...N/...N+A/...N+B/...N+H/...N+C/... N+A+H/...
N+B+H/...N+A+C/...N+B+C/...EB/...EB+A/...EB+B/...EB+N/... EB+H/...EB+C/...EB+N+A/...
EB+N+B/...EB+N+A+H/...EB+N+B+H/.... EB+N+A+C/... EB+N+B+C/.....

Symptoms Noted:_____

Notes:_____

MOLD MIX

AVOID treating on a cloudy, rainy day. Clean up the house well. Keep the house dry. Stay away from leaky bathrooms, old houses etc. Wear freshly washed clothes.

Date treated:_____ Cleared: _____

Combinations needed:.. A/...B/...D/...R/...H/...C/...N/...N+A/...N+B/...N+H/...N+C/... N+A+H/... N+B+H/...N+A+C/...N+B+C/...EB/...EB+A/...EB+B/...EB+N/...EB+H/...EB+C/...EB+N+A/... EB+N+B/...EB+N+A+H/...EB+N+B+H/.... EB+N+A+C/... EB+N+B+C/.....

Symptoms Noted:_____

Notes:_____

DUST MIX and dust mites.

AVOID dusty areas. Clean up the living area before the treatment. Wear a mask for 25 hours.

Date treated:_____ Cleared: _____

Combinations needed:.. A/...B/...D/...R/...H/...C/...N/...N+A/...N+B/...N+H/...N+C/... N+A+H/... N+B+H/...N+A+C/...N+B+C/...EB/...EB+A/...EB+B/...EB+N/...EB+H/...EB+C/...EB+N+A/... EB+N+B/...EB+N+A+H/...EB+N+B+H/.... EB+N+A+C/... EB+N+B+C/.....

Symptoms Noted:_____

Notes:_____

NEWSPAPER/ NEWSPAPER INK

AVOID touching paper goods, newspaper, facial paper, hand towel, pine products, tissue paper etc.

Date treated:_____ Cleared: _____

Combinations needed:.. A/...B/...D/...R/...H/...C/...N/...N+A/...N+B/...N+H/...N+C/... N+A+H/... N+B+H/...N+A+C/...N+B+C/...EB/...EB+A/...EB+B/...EB+N/...EB+H/...EB+C/...EB+N+A/... EB+N+B/...EB+N+A+H/...EB+N+B+H/.... EB+N+A+C/... EB+N+B+C/.....

Symptoms Noted:_____

Notes:_____

MERCURY MIX/AMALGAM

AVOID fish and fish products. avoid mercury products. avoid touching your mouth if you have dental fillings. Wear a pair of gloves for 25 hours.

Date treated:_____   Cleared :_____

Combinations needed:.. A/...B/...D/...R/...H/...C/...N/...N+A/...N+B/...N+H/...N+C/... N+A+H/...
N+B+H/...N+A+C/...N+B+C/...EB/...EB+A/...EB+B/...EB+N/...
EB+H/...EB+C/...EB+N+A/...EB+N+B/...EB+N+A+H/...EB+N+B+H/.... EB+N+A+C/...
EB+N+B+C/

Symptoms Noted:_____

Notes:_____

_____

TREE MIX

AVOID going outdoors. Wear shoes and socks while walking outside. Wear mask and gloves if you are going out.

Date treated:_____   Cleared:_____

Combinations needed:.. A/...B/...D/...R/...H/...C/...N/...N+A/...N+B/...N+H/...N+C/... N+A+H/...
N+B+H/...N+A+C/...N+B+C/...EB/...EB+A/...EB+B/...EB+N/...
EB+H/...EB+C/...EB+N+A/...EB+N+B/...EB+N+A+H/...EB+N+B+H/.... EB+N+A+C/... EB+N+B+C/.....

MEAT MIX

AVOID air conditioned areas, soft plastic products(fluoromethane).

Date treated:_____   Cleared:_____

Combinations needed:.. A/...B/...D/...R/...H/...C/...N/...N+A/...N+B/...N+H/...N+C/... N+A+H/...
N+B+H/...N+A+C/...N+B+C/...EB/...EB+A/...EB+B/...EB+N/...EB+H/...EB+C/...EB+N+A/...
EB+N+B/...EB+N+A+H/...EB+N+B+H/.... EB+N+A+C/... EB+N+B+C/.....

Symptoms Noted:_____

Notes:_____

FLOWER MIX

AVOID going outdoors. Wear shoes and socks while walking outside. Wear mask and gloves if you are going out. Do not smell perfume.

Date treated:_____ Cleared: _____

Combinations needed:.. A/...B/...D/...R/...H/...C/...N/...N+A/...N+B/...N+H/...N+C/... N+A+H/... N+B+H/...N+A+C/...N+B+C/...EB/...EB+A/...EB+B/...EB+N/...EB+H/...EB+C/...EB+N+A/... EB+N+B/...EB+N+A+H/...EB+N+B+H/.... EB+N+A+C/... EB+N+B+C/

Symptoms Noted:_____

Notes:_____

FREON

AVOID air conditioned areas, soft plastic products (fluoromethane).

Date treated:_____ Cleared: _____

Combinations needed:.. A/...B/...D/...R/...H/...C/...N/...N+A/...N+B/...N+H/...N+C/... N+A+H/...N+B+H/...N+A+C/...N+B+C/...EB/...EB+A/...EB+B/...EB+N/... EB+H/...EB+C/...EB+N+A/...EB+N+B/...EB+N+A+H/...EB+N+B+H/.... EB+N+A+C/... EB+N+B+C/

Symptoms Noted:_____

Notes:_____

RADIATION: (sun, microwave, T.V., X-ray, computer).

AVOID sun, T.V., microwave, X-ray & computers for 25 hours.

Date treated:_____ Cleared: _____

Combinations needed:.. A/...B/...D/...R/...H/...C/...N/...N+A/...N+B/...N+H/...N+C/... N+A+H/...N+B+H/...N+A+C/...N+B+C/...EB/...EB+A/...EB+B/...EB+N/...EB+H/... EB+C/...EB+N+A/...EB+N+B/...EB+N+A+H/...EB+N+B+H/.... EB+N+A+C/... EB+N+B+C/....

Symptoms Noted:_____

Notes:_____

CHEMICALS; (soaps, detergents, cleansing chemicals, chlorine, Clorox, bleach).

AVOID contact with the above items for 25 hours. Wash your clothes in plain water prior to treatment.

Date treated:_____ Cleared: _____

Combinations needed:.. A/...B/...D/...R/...H/...C/...N/...N+A/...N+B/...N+H/...N+C/... N+A+H/...

N+B+H/...N+A+C/...N+B+C/...EB/...EB+A/...EB+B/...EB+N/...

EB+H/...EB+C/...EB+N+A/...EB+N+B/...EB+N+A+H/...EB+N+B+H/.... EB+N+A+C/... EB+N+B+C/

Symptoms Noted:_____

Notes:_____

VIRUS MIX: (E.B.V., C.M.V., herpes simplex, herpes zoaster, influenza).

AVOID contact with infected persons for 25 hours. If someone is infected with a virus, treat for the specific sample like herpes zoaster, etc. Also you may take a sample of your own body fluid (saliva, urine, stool, blood, skin tissue, etc.) and treat for it.

YOU MAY EAT everything well cooked and drink boiled, cooled water.

Date treated:_____ Cleared: _____

Combinations needed:.. A/...B/...D/...R/...H/...C/...N/...N+A/...N+B/...N+H/...N+C/... N+A+H/ ...N+B+H/...N+A+C/...N+B+C/...EB/...EB+A/...EB+B/...EB+N/...

EB+H/...EB+C/...EB+N+A/...EB+N+B/...EB+N+A+H/...EB+N+B+H/.... EB+N+A+C/... EB+N+B+C/

Symptoms Noted:_____

Notes:_____

BACTERIA MIX: (Staphylococcus aureus, strepto-coccus (viridans & non-hemolytic), strptococcus, pneumoniae & klebsiella pneumoniae).

AVOID contact with infected surfaces.

YOU MAY EAT everything well cooked and drink boiled, cooled water.

Date treated:_____ Cleared: _____

Combinations needed:.. A/...B/...D/...R/...H/...C/...N/...N+A/...N+B/...N+H/...N+C/... N+A+H/...

N+B+H/...N+A+C/...N+B+C/...EB/...EB+A/...EB+B/...EB+N/...EB+H/...EB+C/...EB+N+A/...

EB+N+B/...EB+N+A+H/...EB+N+B+H/.... EB+N+A+C/... EB+N+B+C/.....

Symptoms Noted:_____

Notes:_____

I.D. (immune deficiency disorder)

Avoid contact with fresh blood from you or anyone else. Avoid meat, fish and eggs.

You may eat cooked vegetables, grains, milk, cheese.

Date treated:_____   Cleared: _____

Combinations needed:.. A/...B/...D/...R/...H/...C/...N/...N+A/...N+B/...N+H/...N+C/... N+A+H/...

N+B+H/...N+A+C/...N+B+C/...EB/...EB+A/...EB+B/...EB+N/...

EB+H/...EB+C/...EB+N+A/...EB+N+B/...EB+N+A+H/...EB+N+B+H/.... EB+N+A+C/... EB+N+B+C/

.....

Symptoms Noted:_____

Notes:_____

_____

HORMONES (estrogen, progesterone, testosterone. check in cases with hot flashes, PMS, hormone imbalances).

AVOID eating or using red meats and products with hormones. If one is able to get the meat from an animal that has never received any hormone, it is OK to eat the red meat from that source. Avoid stimulating your own hormones. Avoid treating during menstrual period.

Date treated:_____   Cleared: _____

Combinations needed:.. A/...B/...D/...R/...H/...C/...N/...N+A/...N+B/...N+H/...N+C/... N+A+H/...N+B+H/...N+A+C/...N+B+C/...EB/...EB+A/...EB+B/...EB+N/...

EB+H/...EB+C/...EB+N+A/...EB+N+B/...EB+N+A+H/...EB+N+B+H/.... EB+N+A+C/... EB+N+B+C/

.....

Symptoms Noted:_____

Notes:_____

_____

SMOKING: (nicotine, tobacco).

 AVOID smoking areas, smoke from cigarettes, clothes and substances made contact with cigarette smoke, banana, malt, cow's milk, potato, tomato and yeast mix. You may wear a mask for 25 hours.

Date treated:_____   Cleared: _____

Combinations needed:.. A/...B/...D/...R/...H/...C/...N/...N+A/...N+B/...N+H/...N+C/... N+A+H/...
N+B+H/...N+A+C/...N+B+C/...EB/...EB+A/...EB+B/...EB+N/...EB+H/...EB+C/...EB+N+A/...
EB+N+B/...EB+N+A+H/...EB+N+B+H/.... EB+N+A+C/... EB+N+B+C/.....

Symptoms Noted:_____

Notes:_____

_____

PERFUME MIX

AVOID perfumed soaps, make-up products, hair sprays, flowers.

You may wear a mask to avoid the smell.

Date treated:_____ Cleared: _____

Combinations needed:.. A/...B/...D/...R/...H/...C/...N/...N+A/...N+B/...N+H/...N+C/... N+A+H/...N+B+H/
...N+A+C/...N+B+C/...EB/...EB+A/...EB+B/...EB+N/...
EB+H/...EB+C/...EB+N+A/...EB+N+B/...EB+N+A+H/...EB+N+B+H/.... EB+N+A+C/... EB+N+B+C/
.....

Symptoms Noted:_____

Notes:_____

WOOD MIX

AVOID contact with woods, things made with woods. You may wear a pair of gloves to avoid contacts with wooden surfaces.

Date treated:_____ Cleared: _____

Combinations needed:.. A/...B/...D/...R/...H/...C/...N/...N+A/...N+B/...N+H/...N+C/... N+A+H/...
N+B+H/...N+A+C/...N+B+C/...EB/...EB+A/...EB+B/...EB+N/...EB+H/...EB+C/...EB+N+A/...
EB+N+B/...EB+N+A+H/...EB+N+B+H/.... EB+N+A+C/... EB+N+B+C/.....

Symptoms Noted:_____

Notes:_____

ITEM TREATED

Date treated:_____ Cleared: _____

Combinations needed:.. A/...B/...D/...R/...H/...C/...N/...N+A/...N+B/...N+H/...N+C/... N+A+H/...N+B+H/...N+A+C/...N+B+C/...EB/...EB+A/...EB+B/...EB+N/...

EB+H/...EB+C/...EB+N+A/...EB+N+B/...EB+N+A+H/...EB+N+B+H/.... EB+N+A+C/... EB+N+B+C/

Symptoms Noted:_____

Notes:_____

_____

ITEM TREATED: _____

AVOID:_____

Datetreated:_____ Cleared: _____

Combinations needed:.. A/...B/...D/...R/...H/...C/...N/...N+A/...N+B/...N+H/...N+C/... N+A+H/...N+B+H/...N+A+C/...N+B+C/...EB/...EB+A/...EB+B/...EB+N/...

EB+H/...EB+C/...EB+N+A/...EB+N+B/...EB+N+A+H/...EB+N+B+H/.... EB+N+A+C/... EB+N+B+C/.....

Symptoms Noted:_____

Notes:_____

_____

ITEM TREATED: _____

AVOID:_____

Date treated:_____ Cleared: _____

ITEMTREATED: _____

Combinations needed:.. A/...B/...D/...R/...H/...C/...N/...N+A/...N+B/...N+H/...N+C/... N+A+H/...N+B+H/...N+A+C/...N+B+C/...EB/...EB+A/...EB+B/...EB+N/...EB+H/...EB+C/...EB+N+A/...EB+N+B/...EB+N+A+H/...EB+N+B+H/.... EB+N+A+C/... EB+N+B+C/.....

Symptoms Noted:_____

Notes:_____

_____

ITEM TREATED: _____

AVOID:_____

Date treated:_____ Cleared: _____ITEM
TREATED: _____

ITEM TREATED: _____

AVOID:_____

Date treated:_____ Cleared: _____

ITEM

TREATED: _____

Combinations needed:.. A/...B/...D/...R/...H/...C/...N/...N+A/...N+B/...N+H/...N+C/... N+A+H/...N+B+H/
...N+A+C/...N+B+C/...EB/...EB+A/...EB+B/...EB+N/...

EB+H/...EB+C/...EB+N+A/...EB+N+B/...EB+N+A+H/...EB+N+B+H/.... EB+N+A+C/... EB+N+B+C/.....

Symptoms Noted:_____

Notes:_____

_____

ITEM TREATED: _____

AVOID:_____

Date treated:_____ Cleared: _____ITEM
TREATED:

Combinations needed:.. A/...B/...D/...R/...H/...C/...N/...N+A/...N+B/...N+H/...N+C/... N+A+H/...N+B+H/
...N+A+C/...N+B+C/...EB/...EB+A/...EB+B/...EB+N/...

EB+H/...EB+C/...EB+N+A/...EB+N+B/...EB+N+A+H/...EB+N+B+H/.... EB+N+A+C/... EB+N+B+C/.....

Symptoms Noted:_____

Notes:_____

_____

ITEM TREATED: _____

AVOID:_____

Date   treated:_____   Cleared:

_____ITEM TREATED:

Combinations needed:.. A/...B/...D/...R/...H/...C/...N/...N+A/...N+B/...N+H/...N+C/... N+A+H/...N+B+H/...N+A+C/...N+B+C/...EB/...EB+A/...EB+B/...EB+N/...

EB+H/...EB+C/...EB+N+A/...EB+N+B/...EB+N+A+H/...EB+N+B+H/.... EB+N+A+C/... EB+N+B+C/.....

Symptoms Noted:_____

Notes:_____

RESOURCES

Lotus Herbs, Inc.
1124 N. Hacienda Blvd.
La Puente, CA 91744, (818) 916-1070,
(Chinese heral formula)

Neuro Emotional Techniques
Dr. Scott Walker
524, 2nd Street,
Encinitas, CA 92024
(760) 944 1030

La Chance Release Method
Dr. Toby Campion, D.C.
8818 W. Olympic Blvd.
Bevery Hills, CA 90211, (310) 273-1221

Kenshin trading Corp.
1815 W. 213th St., #180
Torrance, CA 90501, (310) 212-3199
(Nutritional Products - Garlic, Kelp, Sanza)

Integris Inc.
11 Daytona
Laguna Niguel, CA 92677, (714) 363-9822.
Contact: Dr. David Nelson.
(Nutritional Supplements).

Standard Process Lab.
5621 Palmer Way, Ste.F
Carlsbad, CA 92008, (800) 372-7218
(Nutritional Supplements).

Metagenics, Inc.
971 Calle Negocio
San Clemente, CA 92673, (714) 366-0818

CFIDS Buyers Club
1187 Coast Village Road, #1280
Santa Barbara, CA 93108, (800) 366- 6056

Lab Testing
Great Smoky Mountain Lab
18 A Regent Park Blvd.
Ashville, NC 28806,(800)522-4762

Janice Corp.
198 US High Way 46
Budd Lake, NJ 07828-3001, (800) 526-4237
(Cotton Gloves)

Delta Publishing Co.
6714 Beach Blvd.
Buena Park, CA 90621, Tel. (714) 523-0800
Fax: (714) 523-3068
{ Say Goodbye To Illness}
{Living Pain Free},Web site: naet.com

For NAET seminar please contact:
NAET Seminars
6714 Beach Blvd
Buena Park, CA 90621
(714)523-8900

Bio Meridian, Inc.
1225 E. Fort Union Blvd., Ste #200
Midvale, UT 84047-1882
(801) 561-4707
(Acubase Allergy Testing computer)

For Vetirinary NAET Please call:
Pet Allergy Center
1637 16th st
Santa Monica, CA 90404
(310)-450-2287
www.vetnaet.com

BIBLIOGRAPHY

Austin, Mary. <u>Acupuncture Therapy.</u> New York, 1972.

Beeson, Paul B., M.D. and McDermott, Walsh, M.D., eds. *Textbook of Medicine.* 12th edition, Philadelphia, 1967.

Cerrat, Paul L., "Does Diet Affect the Immune System?" *RN,* Vol. 53, pp. 67-70 (June 1990).

Chaitow, Leon. *The Accupunture Treatment of Pain.* New york: Thorsons Publishers Inc., 1984.

Collins, Douglas, R. M.D. *Illustrated Diagnosis of Systematic Diseases.* Philadelphia, 1972.

Daniels, Lucille, M.A. and Catherine Wothingham, Ph.D. *Muscle Testing Techniques of Manual Examination.* 3rd ed. Philadelphia, 1972

East Asian Medical Studies Society. *Fundamentals of Chinese Medicine.* Brookline: Paraadigm Publications, 1985.

Fazir, Claude A., M.D. *Parents Guide to Allergy in Children.* Garden City: Doubleday & Co. Inc. 1973.

Fulton, Shaton. *The Allergy Self Help Book.* Philadelphia: Rodale Books, 1983.

Fujihara, Ken, and Hays, Nancy. *Common Health Complaints.* Oriental Healing Arts Institute, 1982.

Gabriel, Ingrid. *Herb Identifier and Handbook.* New York: Sterling Publishing Co., Inc., 1980.

Gach, Michael Reed. *Acupppressure's Potent Points.* New York: Bantam Books, 1990.

Golos, Natalie, and Frances. *Coping With Your Allergies.* New York: Simon and Schuster.

Goodheart, George, J. *Applied Kinesiology.* N.P., 1964

Graziano, Joseph. *Footsteps to Better Health,* N.P., 1973

Hsu, Hong-Yen, Ph.D. *Chinese Herb Medicine and Therapy.* Oriental Healing Arts Institute, 1982.

---. *Commonly Used Chinese Herb Formulas with Illustrations.* Oriental Healing Arts Institute, 1982.

---. *Natural Healing With Chinese Herbs.* Oriental Healing Arts Institute, 1982.

Heuns, Him-Che. *Handbook of Chinese Herbs and Formulae.* Vol V. Los Angeles, 1985.

Kennington & Church. *Food Values of Portions Commonly Used.* J.B. Lippincott Company, 1998.

Kirschmann J. D. with L. J. Dunne. *Nutrition Almanac.* 2nd ed. McGraw Hill Book Co. Copyright 1984.

Lawson-Wood, Denis, F.A.C.A. and Joyce Lawson-Wood. *The Five Elements of Acupuncture and Chinese Massage.* 2nd ed. Northamptonshire, 1973.

MacKarness, Richard. *The Hazards of Hidden Allergies.*

Mindell, Earl. *Vitamin Bible.* New York: Warner Books, 1985.

Nambudripad, Devi, S. *Living Pain Free with Acupressure. Delta Publishing Co. Buena Park, Calif, 1997*

Nambudripad, Devi, S. *Say Goodbye to Illness. Delta Publishing Co. Buena Park, Calif, 2nd ed. 1999*

Nambudripad, Devi, S. *The NAET GUIDE BOOK. Delta Publishing Co. Buena Park, Calif, 3rd ed.1998*

Pitchford, Paul. *Healing with Whole Foods.* Berkeley: North Atlantic Books, 1993.

Randolph, Theron, G.,M.D., and Ralph W. Moss, Ph.D. *An Alternative Approach to Allergies.* New York: Lippincott and Conwell, 1980.

Radetsky, Peter. *Allergic to the Twentieth Century.* Boston: Little, Brown and Co., 1997.

Rapp, Doris. *Allergy and Your Family.* New York: Sterling Publishing Co., 1980.

Shanghai College of Traditional Chinese Medicine *Acupuncture, a Comprehensive Text*

Shima, Miky. *The Medical I Ching.* Boulder: Blue Poppy Press, 1992.

Smith, John, H., D.C. *Applied Kinesiology and the Specific Muscle Balancing Technique.*

Case Histories from the Author's private practice, 1984-present.

Index

Symbols

25 HOUR RESTRICTION 17
25-hour clearance 18
25-hour period 3

A

Abdominal Bloating 3, 22
Acid 30
Acupuncture 5, 25
Addictions 8
Air Fresheners 2
Air Purifiers 2
Air-conditioning 10
Alcohol 30, 53
Alcoholism 8, 15
Alkalinity 22
Amalgam 33, 78
Amino Acid 1 29, 48
Amino Acid 2 29, 48
Anaphylaxis 18
Animal 7
Animal Epithelial 32, 78
Animal Fat 29, 47
Ant 78
Anxiety 4
Aroma Therapy 1
Art. Sweeteners 29, 43
Arteriosclerosis 22
Arthritis 11, 22
Aspartame 32, 43
Asthma 5
Atmospheric Changes 9
Autism 22
Auto-immune Disorders 11

B

B Complex 29, 36, 74
Bacteria 11, 12
Bacteria Mix 33, 83
Baking Soda 30, 54
Baking Powder 30, 54
Base 30, 59
Basic Ten 19
Basic Treatments 12
Bee 78
Beet Sugar 32, 74
Berry Mix 31, 74
Bioflavonoids 31, 74
Biotin 31, 37, 74

Bleach 83
Blood 83
Blood Disoders 11
Bluilding Materials. 8
Blurred Vision 4
Body Movements 10
Body Odors 1
Brain Enzymes 22
Brain Fatigue 22
Brain Fog, 22
Brewing Coffee 2
Bronchitis 5, 13
Brown Sugar 32, 74
Buddy System 2
Bupleurum And Dragon Bone Formula 6

C

c.m.v 83
Caffeine 29, 44
Calcium Mix 29, 35
Cancer 11
Candida, 11, 12
Cane Sugar 32, 74
Carpet Deodorizers 2
Carpets 1
Ceramic Cups 8
Cheese Mix 31, 70
Chemical Smells 4
Chemicals 8, 33, 81, 83
Chemotherapy 8
Chicken 31, 34, 74
Chiropractic 5
Chlorides 29, 41
Chlorine 83
Chocolate 29, 44
Cholesterol 23
Choline 31, 38, 74
Chromium 30, 61
Chronic Fatigue 11, 21
Cigarette Smoke 8, 84
Citrus Mix 31, 74
Cleaning Agents 1
Cleansing Chemicals 83
Clearing Practitioner's Allergies 2
Clinic Rules 27
Clorox 2, 83
Cobalt 30, 61
Coffee Brewing 2, 8
Coffee Mix 4, 29, 43
Cold 9, 22

Colitis 10
Colon 22
Colonics 4
Combination Treatments 21
Computer 82
Concrete 8
Concrete Floors 8
Constipation 4, 14
Copper 30, 61
Corn Mix 29, 41
Corn Sugar 32
Cotton 78
Counselling 6
Crohn's Disease 7, 10
Crude Oil 32, 77
Crying Spells 4
Cucumber Mix 31, 72

D

Daily Log 6
Dancing 10
Date Sugar 32, 74
Degenerative Diseases 21
Deodorants 2
Depression 4, 11
Detergents 2, 81, 83
Dextrose 32, 74
Diabetes 8, 11
Diarrhea 4
Diet 24
Digestive Enzymes 13
Distilled Water 12
DNA 22, 30, 58
Doctor's Office 1
Dried Bean Mix 29, 51
Driveways 8
Driving 10
Dryness 10
Dust 2
Dust Mites. 80
Dust Mix 33, 80

E

E.B.V 11, 83
E.Coli 11
Eating Refined Food 19
Eczema 22
Edema 22
Egg Mix 6, 29, 34
Egg White 31, 34, 74
Egg Yolk 31, 34, 74
Electromagnetic Sensitivity 2
Emotion 22
Emotional Allergies 23, 24
Emotional Symptoms 4

Environmental Allergens 74
Environmental Allergies 2
Equal 32, 74
Equilibrium 2
Estrogen 84
Exercise 10, 24, 27

F

Fabric Mix 32, 78
Fabric Softeners 2, 83
Fabrics 8, 12
Feather 34
Fibromyalgia 11, 13, 21
Fibromyalgia 13, 49
Flea 78
Flower Mix 33, 82
Flowers 1, 8
Fluoride 30, 52
Fluoromethane 82
Folic Acid 32, 38, 74
Food Additives 30, 60
Food Allergy 15
Food Coloring 30, 60
Food Combining 11
Food Craving 19
Food Preparation 24
Formaldehyde 2, 8, 32, 77
Foundation 3
Freon 33, 82
Frequency Of The Treatments 15
Fructose 32, 74
Fruit Mix 31, 74
Fumes 77
Fungus 12

G

Gall Bladder 22
Gelatin 13, 30, 53
Germanium 30, 62
Gloves 12, 81
Glucose 32, 74
Gluten Allergy 10
Gold. 62
Good Eating Habits 24
Grain Mix 29, 43
Grass Mix 32, 79, 80
Group 1. 4
Group 2. 5
Group 3. 5
Group 4. 5
Group 5. 5
Gum Mix 30, 54

H

Hair Products 8

Hair Spray 2, 27
Headaches 4, 13, 22
Heart 9, 22
Herbal Extracts 1
Herpes Simplex 83
Herpes Zoaster 83
High Altitude 9
High Blood Pressure 13
High Platelets 11
Honey 32, 74
Hormones 13, 22, 33
Hot Flashes 22, 84
Humidity 9
Hyperactivity 13, 22
Hypersensitivity 15
Hypoglycemia 23

I

I.D 33, 84
Impotency 4
Incense 1
Influenza 83
Inositol 31, 38, 74
Insect Mix 32, 78
Insomnia 14, 15
Intestinal Disorders 10
Iodine 30, 64
Iron Mix 29, 39
Irritability 13, 22
Irritable Bowel Syndrome 7, 10
Itching 4
Items To Treat Together 33

J

Jogging 10
Juice Fast 19

K

Kidney 22

L

L-Glutamine 6
La Chance Release Techniques 6
Lactose 32, 72
Lead 30, 63
Leather 27
Lecithin 31, 70
Leukemia 11
Liquid Paper 77
Liver 5, 22
Living Pain Free With Acupressure 12
Lotus Herbs 5, 6
Loud Noise 2

Low Altitude 9
Low Libido 4
Low White Blood Cells 11
Lungs 22

M

Magnesium 30, 64
Malathion 32, 76
Maltose 32, 74
Manganese 30, 64
Manic Disorders 13
Maple Sugar 32
Marbles 8
Massage 24
Meat Mix 32, 81
Melon Mix 31, 76
Mercury 12, 33,
Mercury Mix 81
Microwave 82
Microwave Oven 2
Milk Allergy 8
Milk Mix 31, 70
Mineral Mix 29, 40
Modified Starch 31, 73
Mold 2, 12
Mold Mix 33, 80
Molybdenum 30, 64, 65
Mood Swings 4
MRT 2, 8
MSG 32, 75
Muscle Aches 14

N

N.A.R.F. 2
NAET 1, 2, 11, 12
NAET practitioners 2
Nail Polish 8
Nambudripad's Allergy Elimination Techniques 1
Nambudripad's Allergy Research Foundation 2
Nausea 4
Neuro Emotional Techniques 6
New Clothes 77
Newsletter 2
Newspaper 2, 8, 33, 77, 78, 80
Nicotine 84
Normal Reaction After Treatments 3
Nut Mix 1 29, 45
Nut Mix 2 29, 45

O

Obesity 23
Obsession 4
Onion Mix 31, 71
Order Of Treatments 14
Osteoporosis 22

Other Allergens 31, 74
Overeating, 15

P

P.M.S 22, 84
PABA 8, 31, 38, 74
Paint Thinner 77
Paints 1, 8
Pancreas 22
Paper 33, 78
Parasites 11
Penicillin 8
Pepper Mix 31, 72
Perfume 2, 27, 33, 85
Pesticides 13, 32, 76
Phenylalanine 6
Phosphorus 30, 65
Physical Symptoms 3, 4
Pituitrophin 59
Plastics 32, 76
Pneumonia 13, 22
Pollen Mix 33, 79
Polyester 78
Poor Concentration 13
Poor Memory 13
Popcorn 2, 8, 24
Potassium 30, 65
Potato Mix 31, 71
Pregnant Women 25
Preparation For Treatments 12
Pressed Wood 77
Progesterone 84
Psychiatrists 5
PT 30

R

Radiation 8, 33, 79, 82
Raynaud's Disease 23
Reactions During Naet 4
Record Keeping 26
Red wine 32
Rice Sugar/ Corn Sugar/ Honey 32, 74
 Lactose/ Maple Sug 32, 74
Ringing In The Ears 4
RNA 22, 30, 58
RNA/DNA 21, 58
rowing 10
running 10

S

Saccharine 32, 74
Sailing 110
saliva , 11, 83
Salt, 4
Salt Mix 29, 41

Sauna 5
Say Goodbye To Illness 1
Scleroderma 23
Selenium 30, 67
Serotonin 22, 30, 59
Serum Triglycerides 22
Shell Fish Mix 29, 49
Shower 27
Silver 30, 66
Sinusitis 13, 15
Sleep Disorders 13
Smoking 8, 27, 84
Smoking /Nicotine 33, 84
Soaps 83
Sorbitol 32, 74
Aspartame/ Saccharine 32, 74
Sweet 'N' Low/ Equal 32, 74
Soybean Mix 31, 68
Spice Mix 1 29, 46
Spice Mix 2 29, 46
Spices 4
Spider 78
Staphylo-coccus 83
Stomach 22
Stomach Acids 13, 22, 58
Strepto-coccus 83
Sugar 4, 12, 22, 23
Sugar Craving 22
Sugar Mix 29, 39
Suicidal Thoughts 4
Sulfites 22
Sulfur 30, 68
Sun 82
Supplements 20
Support Group 3
Surrogate Treatment 7
Sweet 'N' Low 32, 74

T

T. V. 82
Tachycardia 4
Tennis, 10
Testosterone 84
Tetracycline 33, 34, 74
Tiles 8
Tobacco 84
Tomato Mix 31, 70
Trace Minerals 13, 40
Treating For Clouds 9
Tree Mix 33, 81
Turkey 29, 51, 59
Tyrosine 6

U

Ulcerative Colitis 7

Unusual Conditions 26
Urine 11, 83

V

Vanadium 30, 67
Varicose Vein 4
Vegetable Fats 29, 47
Vegetable Mix 29, 54
Vinegar Mix 31, 74
Virus 11, 12, 33, 83
Virus Mix 33, 83
Vitality Formula 5
Vitamin A 29, 40
Vitamin B1 31, 36, 74
Vitamin B2 31, 36, 74
Vitamin B3 31, 36, 74
Vitamin B4 31, 36, 74
Vitamin B5 31, 36, 74
Vitamin B6 31, 37, 74
Vitamin B12 8, 31, 37, 74
Vitamin B13 32, 37, 74
Vitamin B15 32, 37, 74
Vitamin B17 32, 37, 74
Vitamin C Mix 29, 35
Vitamin D 30, 55
Vitamin E 30, 55
Vitamin F 30, 56
Vitamin K 30, 56
Vitamin P 30, 57
Vitamin T 30, 57

W

Walking 10
Wall Paper 2
Water Fast 5
Weakness Of The Knees 8
Weed Mix 33, 79
Wheat Mix 31, 72
Whey 29, 50
White Wine 32, 75
White Wine/ Red Wine 32, 75
Whiten-all 30, 52
Wood 27
Wood Furniture 8
Wood Mix 33, 85

X

X-ray 82

Y

Yeast Mix 29, 42
Yeast/ Candida 11, 42
Yogurt 29, 50

Z

Zinc 31, 68

NOTES

NOTES

NOTES

NOTES